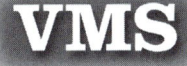

VISUAL MNEMONICS
FOR
BEHAVIORAL SCIENCES

VMS

Visual Mnemonics for Microbiology and Immunology

Visual Mnemonics for Pharmacology

Visual Mnemonics for Pathology

Visual Mnemonics for Physiology and Related Anatomy

Visual Mnemonics for Biochemistry

Visual Mnemonics for Behavioral Sciences

VMS

VISUAL MNEMONICS FOR BEHAVIORAL SCIENCES

LAURIE L. MARBAS, M.D., M.B.A.
Resident, Department of Family Medicine
Texas Tech University Health Sciences Center
Lubbock, Texas

ERIN CASE, M.D.
Resident, Department of Family Medicine
Texas Tech University Health Sciences Center
Lubbock, Texas

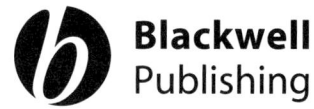

Blackwell Publishing

© 2004 by Blackwell Publishing

Blackwell Publishing, Inc.,
   350 Main Street, Malden, Massachusetts 02148-5018, USA
Blackwell Publishing Ltd,
   9600 Garsington Road, Oxford OX4 2DQ, UK
Blackwell Science Asia Pty Ltd,
   550 Swanston Street, Carlton, Victoria 3053, Australia

All rights reserved. No part of this publication may be reproduced in any form or by any electronic or mechanical means, including information storage and retrieval systems, without permission in writing from the publisher, except by a reviewer who may quote brief passages in a review.

03 04 05 06 5 4 3 2 1
ISBN: 1-4051-0364-7

Library of Congress Cataloging-in-Publication Data

Marbas, Laurie L.
   Visual mnemonics for behavioral sciences /
   Laurie L. Marbas, Erin Case.
      p. ; cm. — (Visual mnemonics series)
Includes index.
   ISBN 1-4051-0364-7 (pbk.)
      1. Psychiatry—Outlines, syllabi, etc.
      2. Psychiatry—Charts, diagrams, etc. 3. Mnemonics.
   [DNLM: 1. Mental Disorders—Terminology—English.
   2. Association Learning. WM 15 M312v 2003] I. Case, Erin.
   II. Title. III. Series.
RC457.2.M37 2003
616.89′002′02—dc22   2003015292

A catalogue record for this title is available from the British Library

Acquisitions: Beverly Copland
Development: Kate Heinle
Production: Jennifer Kowalewski
Cover design: Meral Dabcovich
Interior design: Shawn Girsberger
Typesetter: International Typesetting and Composition, in India
Printed and bound by Sheridan Books, in Michigan

For further information on Blackwell Publishing, visit our website: www.blackwellpublishing.com

Notice: The indications and dosages of all drugs in this book have been recommended in the medical literature and conform to the practices of the general community. The medications described do not necessarily have specific approval by the Food and Drug Administration for use in the diseases and dosages for which they are recommended. The package insert for each drug should be consulted for use and dosage as approved by the FDA. Because standards for usage change, it is advisable to keep abreast of revised recommendations, particularly those concerning new drugs.

CONTENTS

1. DISORDERS ASSOCIATED WITH COGNITIVE IMPAIRMENT
 Delirium   2
 Dementia   4

2. PSYCHOTIC DISORDERS
 Schizophrenia   6
 Schizoaffective Disorder   8
 Delusional Disorder   10

3. MOOD DISORDERS
 Major Depressive Disorder   12
 Dysthymic Disorder   14
 Bipolar I and Bipolar II   16
 Cyclothymic Disorder   18

4. PERSONALITY DISORDERS
 Cluster A Personality Disorders   20
 Cluster B Personality Disorders   22
 Cluster C Personality Disorders   24

5. ANXIETY DISORDERS
 Generalized Anxiety Disorder   26
 Obsessive-Compulsive Disorder (OCD)   28
 Post-Traumatic Stress Disorder   30
 Panic Disorder   32

6. SOMATOFORM DISORDERS, FACTITIOUS DISORDERS, AND MALINGERING
 Somatization Disorder   34
 Conversion Disorder   36
 Hypochondriasis   38
 Body Dysmorphic Disorder   40
 Pain Disorder   42
 Factitious Disorder   44
 Malingering   46

7. SUBSTANCE ABUSE
 Alcohol Abuse and Dependence   48
 Alcohol Intoxication   50
 Amphetamine Intoxication   52
 Cannabis Intoxication   54
 Cocaine Intoxication   56
 Hallucinogen Intoxication   58
 Opioid Intoxication   60
 Sedative, Hypnotic, or Anxiolytic Intoxication   62

8. EATING DISORDERS
 Anorexia Nervosa   64
 Bulimia Nervosa   66

9. DISSOCIATIVE DISORDERS
 Dissociative Amnesia   68
 Dissociative Fugue   70
 Dissociative Identity Disorder   72
 Depersonalization Disorder   74

10. PSYCHOSEXUAL DISORDERS
 Sexual Response Cycle   76
 Sexual Dysfunctions   78

11. PARAPHILIAS
 Paraphilias   80

12. PHOBIAS
 Agoraphobia   82
 Social Phobia   84

13. DISORDERS OF CHILDHOOD AND ADOLESCENCE
 Attention Deficit Disorder   86
 Tourette's Disorder   88
 Autistic Disorder   90
 Asperger's Disorder   92
 Rett's Disorder   94
 Oppositional Defiant Disorder   96
 Conduct Disorder   98

14. PSYCHOTHERAPIES
 Psychoanalysis   100
 Behavioral Theory   102
 Behavioral and Cognitive Therapies   104

15. SLEEP AND SLEEP DISORDERS
 Stages of Sleep   106
 Dyssomnias   108
 Parasomnias   110

16. EGO DEFENSES
 Altruism, Repression, Humor, Sublimation, Suppression   112
 Acting Out, Splitting, Regression, Denial, Rationalization, Reaction Formation   114
 Projection, Displacement, Identification, Intellectualization, Dissociation, Undoing   116

APPENDICES
   A. Terms to Understand and Remember   118
   B. Biopsychosocial Assessment   119
   C. Erikson's Life Cycle Stages   120
   D. Medical Ethics and Communication   121
   E. Epidemiology and Biostatistics   122

INDEX   125

PREFACE

Visual Mnemonics is a study tool that aids in quickly learning and memorizing material presented in behavioral sciences. Two significant features of *Visual Mnemonics* are the long-term retention of material and the increased rate of learning. This allows the student more time to study the fraction of material not covered in the *Visual Mnemonics* book.

These illustrations were created to assist in my own studying because I was always short on time to efficiently memorize facts, and then I was frustrated because I couldn't remember them longer than an hour after the test. As a mom of three small children, my time for studying is limited and must be high-yield 100% of the time. These illustrations allowed me, and many classmates, to do that. Several classmates stated to me that their grades improved 10 points from one exam to the next. Also, we all agree that long-term retention is incredible compared to traditional study methods of memorizing from lists or notecards.

I have attempted to combine as many pertinent facts and functions into the illustrations as possible. This book is not meant to be an end-all to your studying, but it certainly can provide an efficient and more stimulating method of studying the material that is contained in the illustrations.

Some tips on using the pictures: Look at them after you have read your class notes, or gone to class, and so on. Then you will know what material is not covered in this book and what material is deemed important in your particular curriculum. Also, write on them, color them, redraw them, add your own drawings to them—the more the illustrations are manipulated, the more information will be retained in long-term memory. Some students rewrite notes to study, and you can write this information in the book. It will be concise, and everything will be in one place for you.

ACKNOWLEDGMENTS

Throughout my medical education I have been blessed with many opportunities, which I thank the Lord for every day. A special thank you must go to my grandmother, Maxine Turner, for watching my three children while I attended my first two years of medical school. Without her, none of this would have been possible. My husband, Patrick Marbas, also deserves a tremendous debt of gratitude for making many sacrifices for me, including driving 100 miles one-way to work every day, so that I could attend medical school. In addition, much love to my three beautiful children, Emily, Jonathan, and Gabriel, for playing quietly while I studied and giving me hugs of encouragement when I needed it the most.

A special thank you to Erin Case for her friendship and dedication to our project during difficult and trying times.

—Laurie Marbas

I would love to thank my beautiful family for helping me, while putting up with me at the same time. My husband, Jay, has been a triumph of love and support while I worked on this book. I truly thank him for helping keep me sane. He also gives great back rubs. I would also like to thank my sweet three-year-old daughter, Violet, who supports me with hugs, kisses, and happiness. A special thanks to my beautiful mom, Christine, for her love and all the babysitting. A thanks goes to my dad, Roger, for inspiring me to go into medicine. A world of thanks goes to my best friend ever, Laurie, for being the best listener and chauffeur. Thank you, Laurie, for giving me this great opportunity.

—Erin Case

1. Disorders Associated with Cognitive Impairment

COGNITIVE DISORDERS: DELIRIUM

- DSM-IV-TR criteria include:
  - Characterized by a disturbance of consciousness, cognition, and attention
  - Develops over a short period (hours to days)
  - Changes throughout the course of a day
  - Change in cognition is not caused by dementia
- Classification of delirium
  - General medical condition
  - Substance intoxication or withdrawal
  - Multifactorial
- Occurs in 10% to 15% of hospitalized patients, with increased rates in elderly
- Causes of delirium
  - General medical conditions:
    - Postsurgical
    - Metabolic disturbances include hyponatremia, hypoglycemia, hypoxia, hypercapnia, hypercalcemia
    - Infectious causes include urinary tract infections, meningitis, pneumonia, and sepsis
    - Endocrine causes include hypothyroidism and hyperthyroidism
    - Head trauma
    - Seizures
    - Thiamine deficiency
    - Substance-induced causes include alcohol, benzodiazepines, opioids, hallucinogens, stimulants, and sedatives
    - Substance withdrawal causes include alcohol, benzodiazepines, and barbiturates
    - Toxic causes include anticholinergic, carbon monoxide, or organophosphate toxicity
- Clinical features of delirium:
  - Onset develops over hours to days
    ⇒ clock
  - Course changes within a day and may include periods of both lucidity and confusion
    lucidity ⇒ moon
    confusion ⇒ ???
  - Consciousness is impaired
    ⇒ eye closed
  - Attention is impaired
  - Cognition is impaired, including memory, language, and orientation
    ⇒ where am I?
  - Hallucinations may occur
  - Disturbed sleep-wake cycles
    ⇒ eye closed/open
  - Psychomotor agitation (falling, pulling out IVs and catheters)
    ⇒ angry face
  - Sundowning (worsening of symptoms at night)
    ⇒ sunset
  - Medical and/or substance-related causes
  - Resolution within hours to weeks
- Treatment includes:
  - Treating the underlying cause
  - Haloperidol is often used to treat agitation and may be given oral, IM, or IV
    ⇒ halo
  - Lorazepam (Ativan) may also be used for agitation and is available oral, IM, or IV
  - Clocks and calendars to aid in orientation
  - Restraints may be used to prevent injury to self or others

Delirium

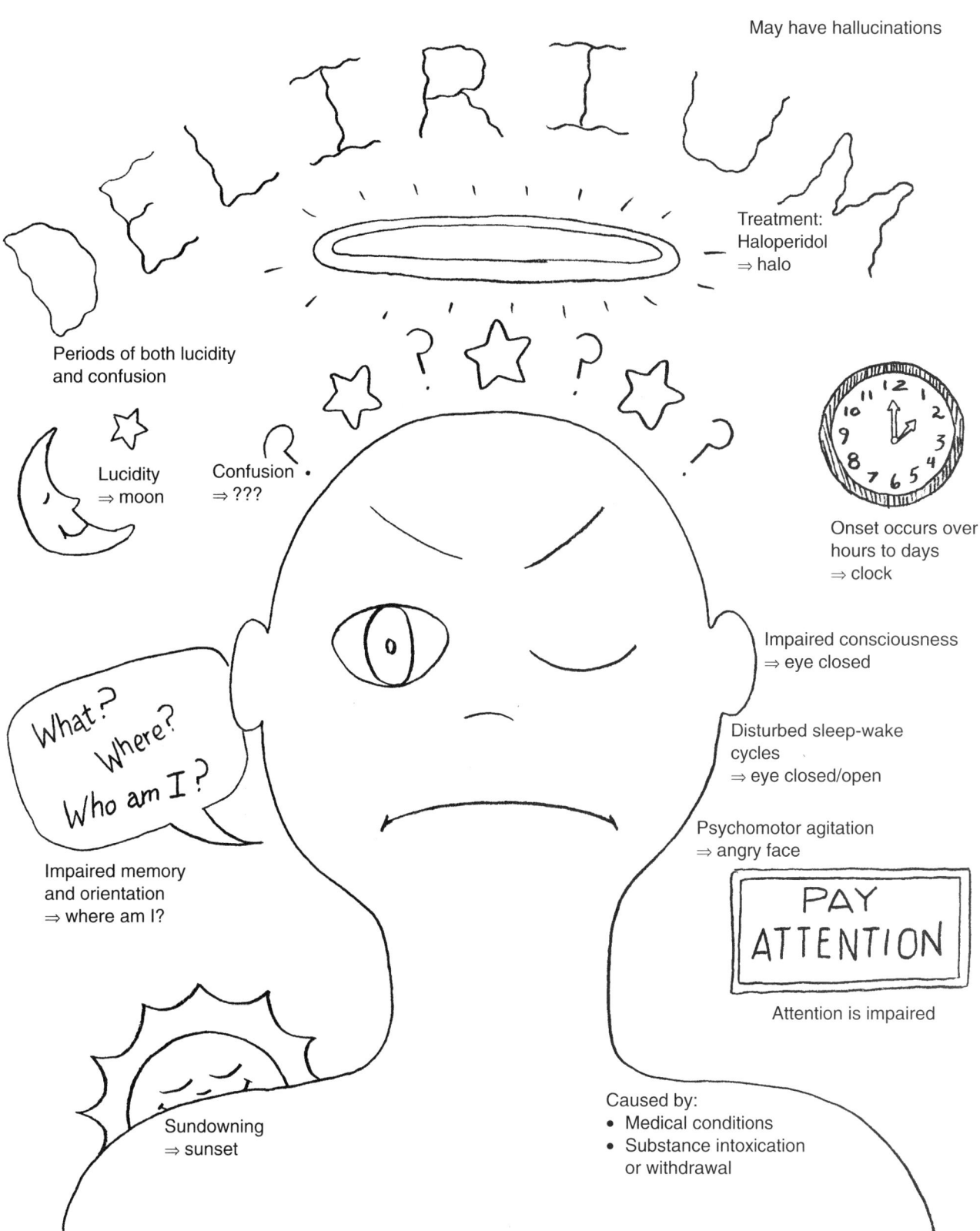

1. Disorders Associated with Cognitive Impairment

COGNITIVE DISORDERS: DEMENTIA

- DSM-IV-TR criteria include:
  - Characterized by memory impairment and other cognitive deficits
  - One or more of the following:
    - Aphasia: Language disturbance
    - Agnosia: Difficulty identifying objects
    - Apraxia: Difficulty carrying out purposeful movements
    - Difficulty planning and carrying out tasks
  - Causes impairment in social and occupational functioning
  - Changes not caused by delirium
- Occurs in about 3% of people older than age 65, and increases to 20% of those older than age 85
- Causes of dementia:
  - Alzheimer's disease
    ⇒ high in the Alps
    - Most common cause of dementia, 50% to 60% of all cases
    - Death occurs 8 to 10 years after onset
    - Cortical atrophy, amyloid plaques, neurofibrillary tangles, decrease in acetylcholine in cerebral cortex
    - Increased incidence in Down syndrome
  - Vascular dementia
    - Second most common cause of dementia
    - Vascular causes include multiple infarcts, congestive heart failure (CHF), collagen vascular diseases, subacute bacterial endocarditis
    - Focal neurologic findings
    - Onset may be abrupt or slowly progressive
  - Parkinson's disease
    ⇒ park
    - Depigmentation of substantia nigra
    - Degeneration of dopaminergic neurons
    - Resting pill-rolling tremor, expressionless facies, shuffling gait, slowed voluntary movements, bradyphrenia (slowed thinking)
  - Huntington's disease
    ⇒ hunting gun
    - Autosomal-dominant defect on chromosome 4
    - Atrophy of caudate nucleus
    - Choreiform movements
  - Pick's disease
    - Atrophy of frontal and temporal lobes
    - Pick bodies
    - More common in women
  - Creutzfeldt-Jakob disease
    - Possible prion transmission
    - Spongiform encephalopathy present
    - Triad consists of dementia, myoclonus, and abnormal EEG
  - HIV-related dementia
    HIV ⇒ hive
    - Caused by the direct effect of the human immunodeficiency virus (HIV) on the brain
    - Affects the white matter and cerebral cortex
  - Head trauma
    - Deficits are stable and usually do not progress
  - Other neurologic causes of dementia include:
    - Brain tumors, normal-pressure hydrocephalus, cerebral hypoxia, seizures, and multiple sclerosis
    - Nutrition deficiencies of folate, vitamin B_{12}, or thiamine can cause dementia that may be reversible
    - Infectious causes of dementia include HIV, encephalitis, cryptococcal meningitis, and neurosyphilis
    - Other medical causes of dementia include hepatic encephalopathy, hypothyroidism, hyperparathyroidism, and Wilson's disease
- Clinical features of dementia:
  - Onset develops over weeks to years
    ⇒ calendar
  - Course is stable within a day
  - Course may progress over weeks to years
  - Memory impairment
  - Orientation and language are impaired
  - Executive functioning is impaired (planning and carrying out tasks)
  - May have hallucinations and delusions
  - Disturbed sleep-wake cycles
  - Mood disturbances
  - Psychomotor agitation
    ⇒ angry face
  - Short-term memory greatly affected
  - Difficulty recalling names and recognizing objects
  - Difficulty learning new material
  - May have difficulty with activities of daily living
  - Poor insight and judgment
  - Eventually patients may become depressed, incontinent, and bedridden
  - Dementia may be reversible or partially reversible with nutritional deficiencies, hydrocephalus, and neurosyphilis
- Pseudodementia can be distinguished from dementia
  - Pseudodementia is associated with depression, and mood disturbances are great
  - In pseudodementia, patients frequently answer "I don't know" but may eventually answer correctly if pressured
- Treatment includes:
  - Treating the underlying cause
  - Treatment of Alzheimer's disease
    - Donepezil (Aricept) inhibits acetylcholinesterase to increase levels of acetylcholine in the central nervous system (CNS), which improves cognitive functioning
    - Tacrine (Cognex) is also an acetylcholinesterase inhibitor; AST and ACT must be monitored because of hepatotoxicity
  - Low doses of high-potency antipsychotics are used to treat agitation and hallucinations
  - Low doses of benzodiazepines are used to treat anxiety, insomnia, and agitation
  - Selective serotonin reuptake inhibitors (SSRIs) are used to treat depression

Dementia

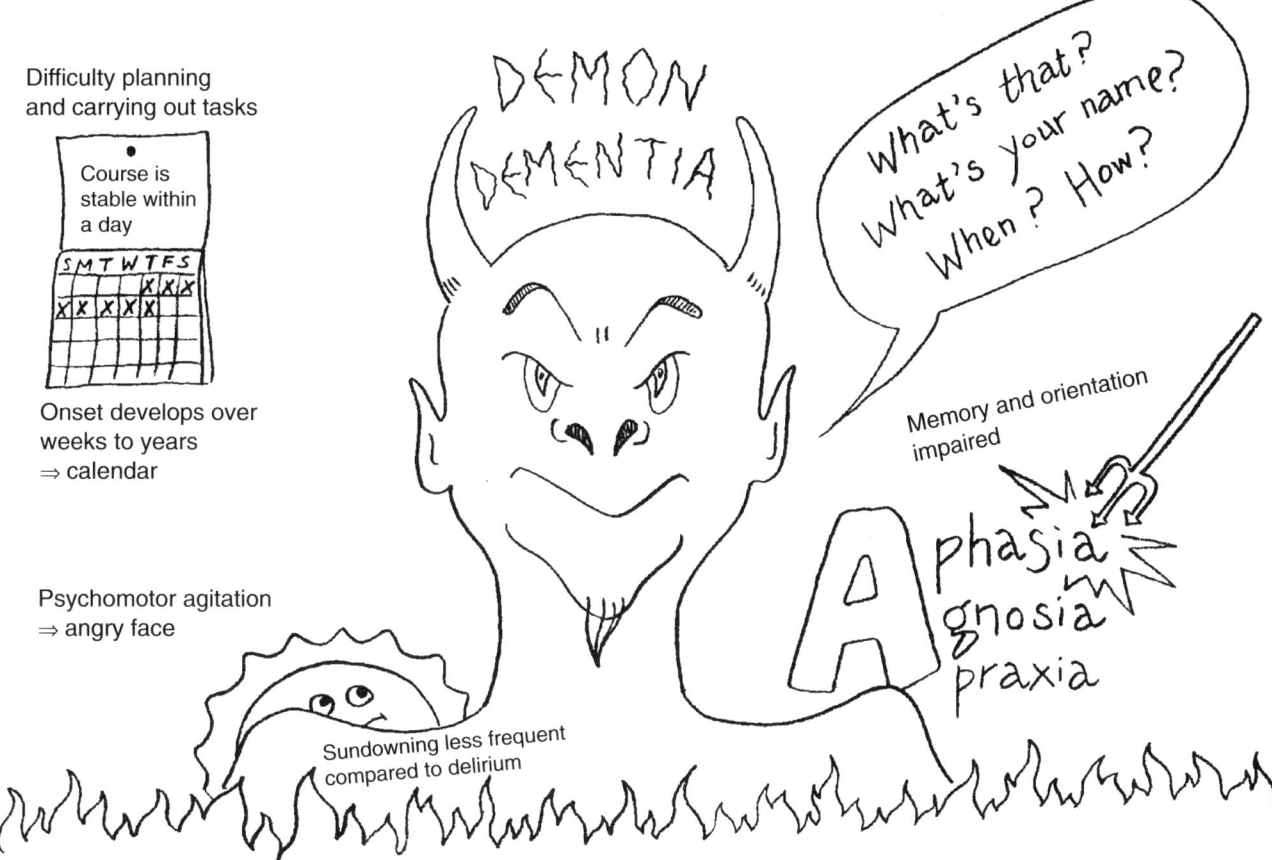

Specific causes of dementia:

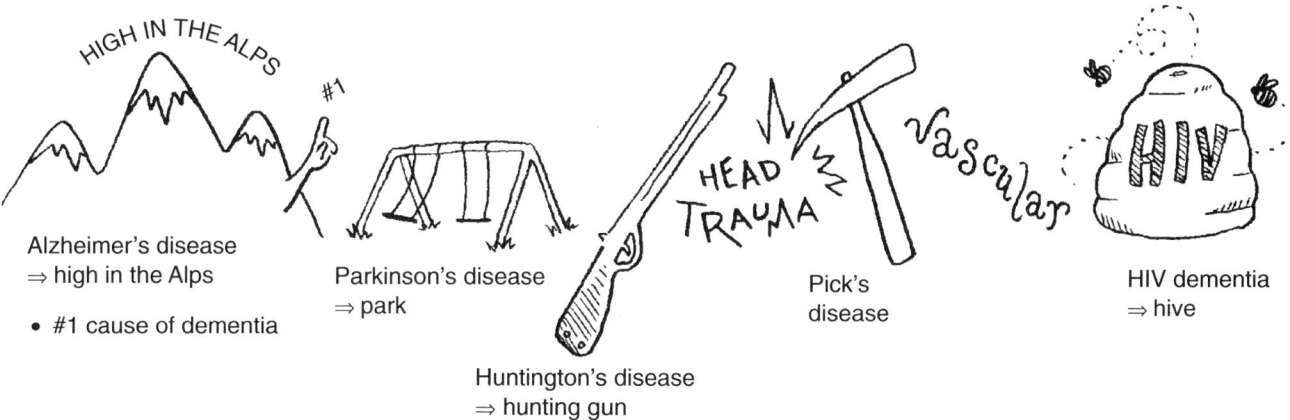

2. Psychotic Disorders

SCHIZOPHRENIA AND SCHIZOPHRENIFORM DISORDER

■ SCHIZOPHRENIA

- Etiology: Defect in dopaminergic system
- Two or more psychotic symptoms listed below present for at least one month:
  - Delusions (**false beliefs** inconsistent with external environment and individual's experience)
  - Hallucinations (**false perceptions** inconsistent with external stimuli; can involve auditory, visual, olfactory, and tactile senses)
  - Disorganized speech (incoherent)
  - Disorganized or catatonic behavior
  - Negative symptoms (affective flattening, alogia, avolition, lack of motivation)

  *Only one symptom above required for diagnosis if bizarre delusions present; hallucinations consisting of one continual voice or voices speak to one another.
- Impairment of social or occupational functioning
- Duration of illness must be at least 6 months
- Subclassifications:
  - Catatonic: Motor abnormalities including excessive movements or rigidity; also posturing, echolalia, or echopraxia
  - Disorganized: Flat affect and disorganized speech or behavior
  - Paranoid: Preoccupation with auditory hallucinations or delusions
- Affects younger individuals in late teens, twenties, and thirties
- Positive symptoms preclude a more favorable prognosis than if patient has a majority of negative symptoms
  - Positive symptoms: Delusions, hallucinations, strange behavior, and loose associations
  - Negative symptoms: Lack of motivation, flat affect, thought blocking, and social withdrawal
- Treatment: Haloperidol for positive symptoms and other neuroleptics, also long-term supportive psychotherapy

■ SCHIZOPHRENIFORM DISORDER

- Same symptoms as schizophrenia noted above; however, symptoms last longer than one month but less than 6 months
- Only approximately 30% of patients recover fully within the six-month period, and the rest develop schizophrenia

Schizophrenia

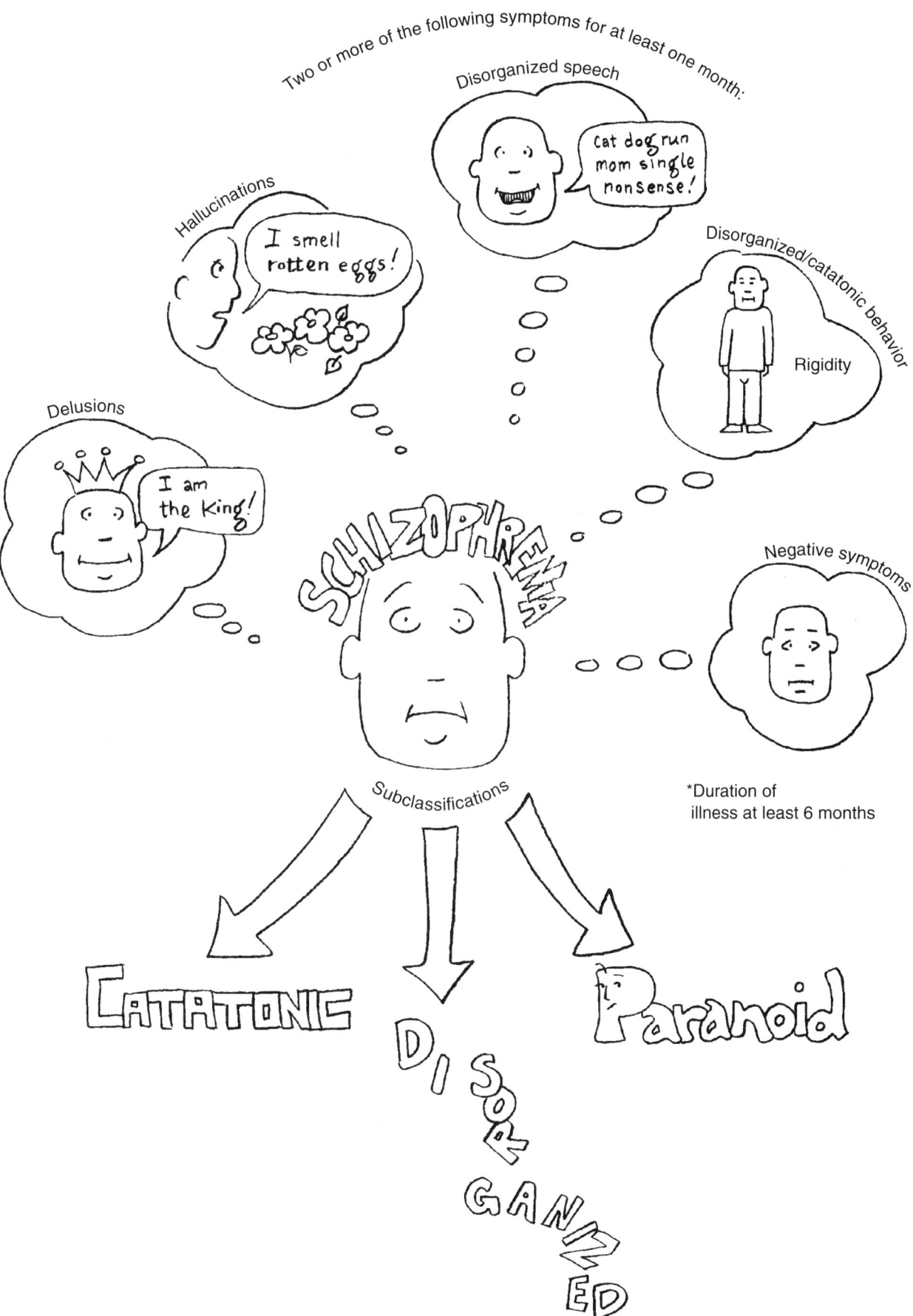

2. Psychotic Disorders

SCHIZOAFFECTIVE DISORDER

- Patient has depressive or manic symptoms with psychotic symptoms
- When the patient is not in depressed or manic state, residual schizophrenic-like symptoms persist (if psychotic symptoms only present with mania/depression, then patient should be considered for diagnosis of primary mood disorder with psychotic features)
- During illness, delusions/hallucinations have occurred at least 2 weeks without mood symptoms
- Two types:
  - Bipolar: Includes manic or mixed episodes
  - Depressive: Includes only major depressive episodes

Schizoaffective Disorder

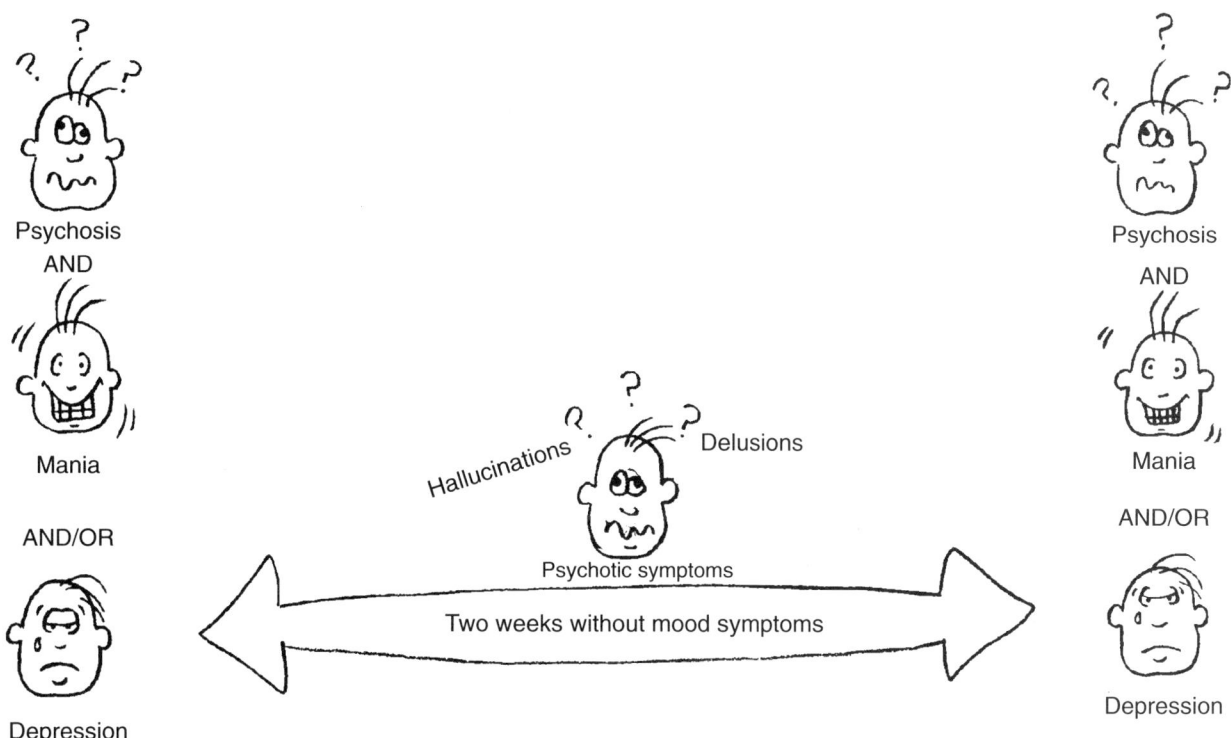

2. Psychotic Disorders

DELUSIONAL DISORDER

- Nonbizarre delusions lasting at least one month
- Schizophrenia criteria are not met
- Social or occupational functioning is not impaired
- Hallucinations may be present if part of delusional theme
- Types:
  - Grandiose: Delusions of inflated worth or power
  - Persecutory: Delusions of being treated malevolently
  - Erotomanic: Delusions that another individual of higher status is in love with him or her
  - Jealous: Delusions that sexual partner is unfaithful
  - Somatic: Delusions of physical defects or illness
  - Mixed: More than one mentioned above is present and none dominate
  - Unspecified
- Usually refractory to treatment

Delusional Disorder

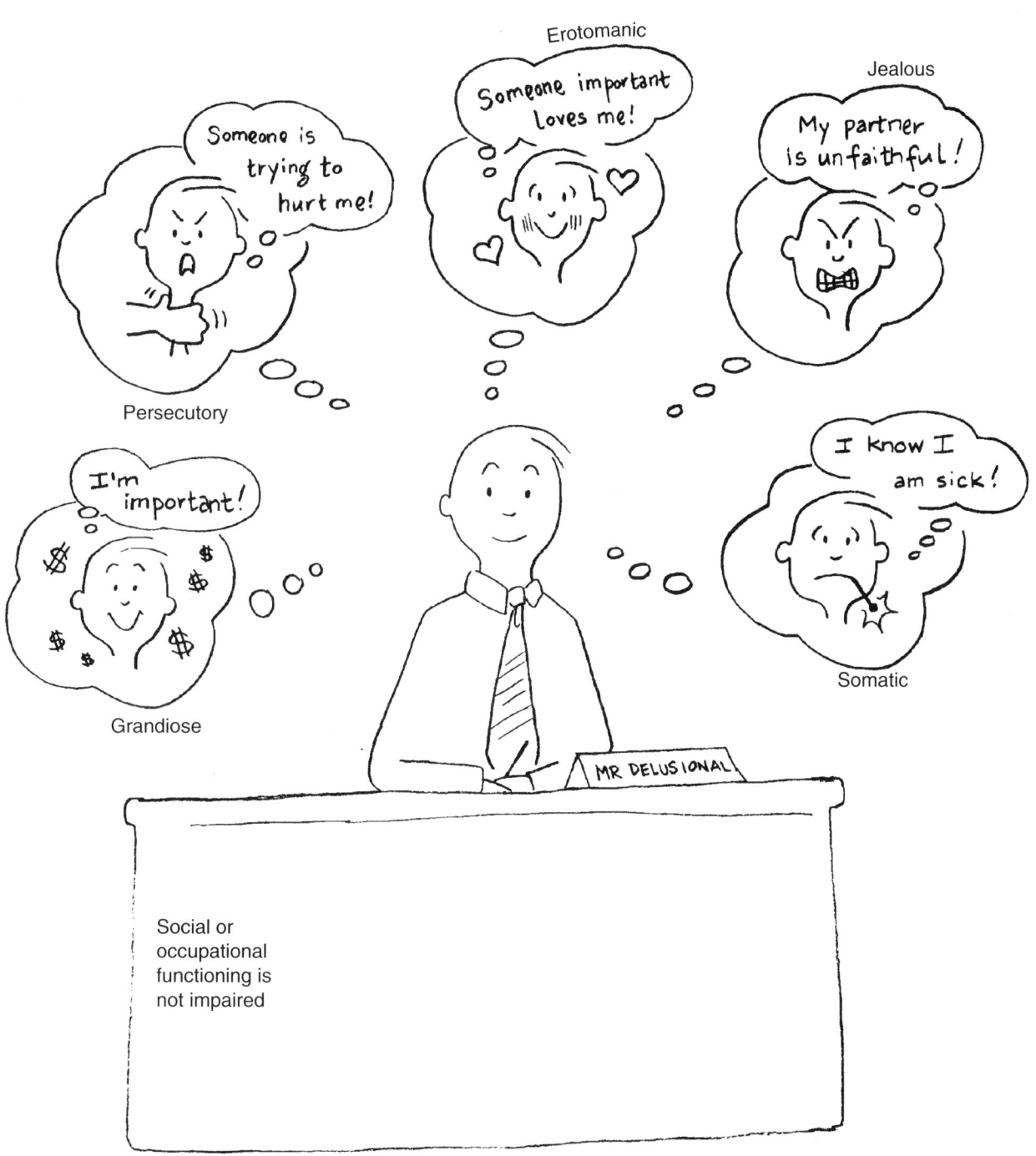

3. Mood Disorders

MAJOR DEPRESSIVE DISORDER (AS DEFINED BY DSM-IV-TR)

- Major depressive episode
  - Five of the following during a two-week period, including a depressed mood, or loss of interest or pleasure
    - Depressed mood most of day, nearly every day
    - Decreased interest or pleasure in activities nearly every day
    - Unintentional weight loss or weight gain
    - Sleep disturbances (insomnia or hypersomnia)
    - Psychomotor agitation or retardation
    - Fatigue nearly every day
    - Feeling worthless or inappropriate guilt
    - Difficulty concentrating
    - Recurrent thoughts of death
- Major depressive disorder
  - Two or more major depressive episodes with at least a consecutive two-month interval between them
  - Episodes are not accounted for by other disorders, and there has never been a manic, mixed, or hypomanic episode
- Treatment
  - Hospitalization may be required
  - Antidepressant therapy should be started; selective serotonin reuptake inhibitors (SSRIs) would be safe in case of overdose

Major Depressive Disorder

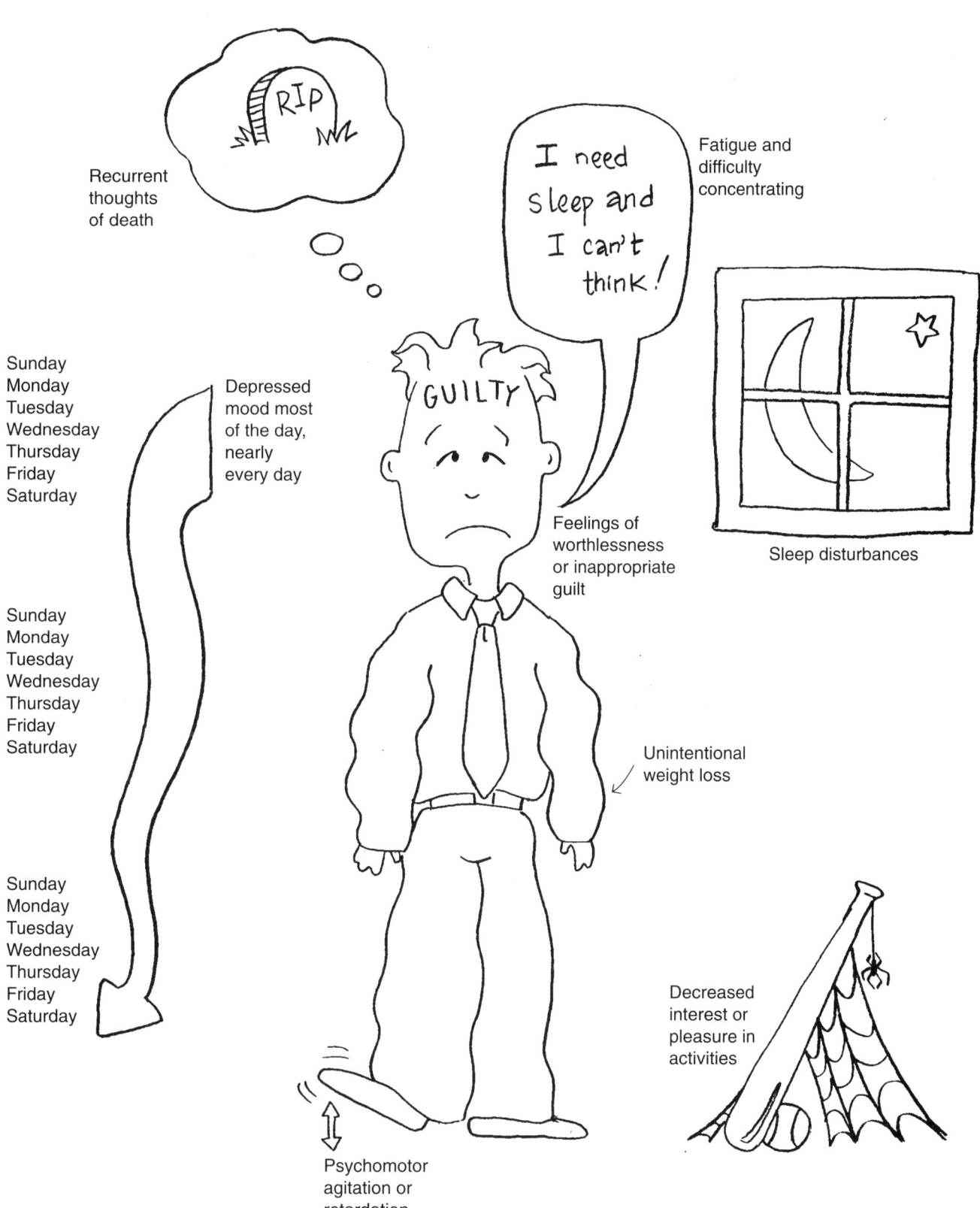

3. Mood Disorders

NOTES

DYSTHYMIC DISORDER (AS DEFINED BY DSM-IV-TR)

- Depressed mood most of day, more days than not for two years
- While depressed, two or more of the following are present:
  - Increase or decrease in appetite
  - Sleep disturbances (insomnia or hypersomnia)
  - Fatigue
  - Low self-esteem
  - Difficulty concentrating
  - Feeling hopeless
- During two-year period, person never went without symptoms for more than two months
- During two years, there was never a major depressive episode
- Episodes are not accounted for by other disorders, and there has never been a manic, mixed, or hypomanic episode
- Treatment should include insight-oriented psychotherapy and behavioral therapy; a trial of antidepressants may also be beneficial

Dysthymic Disorder

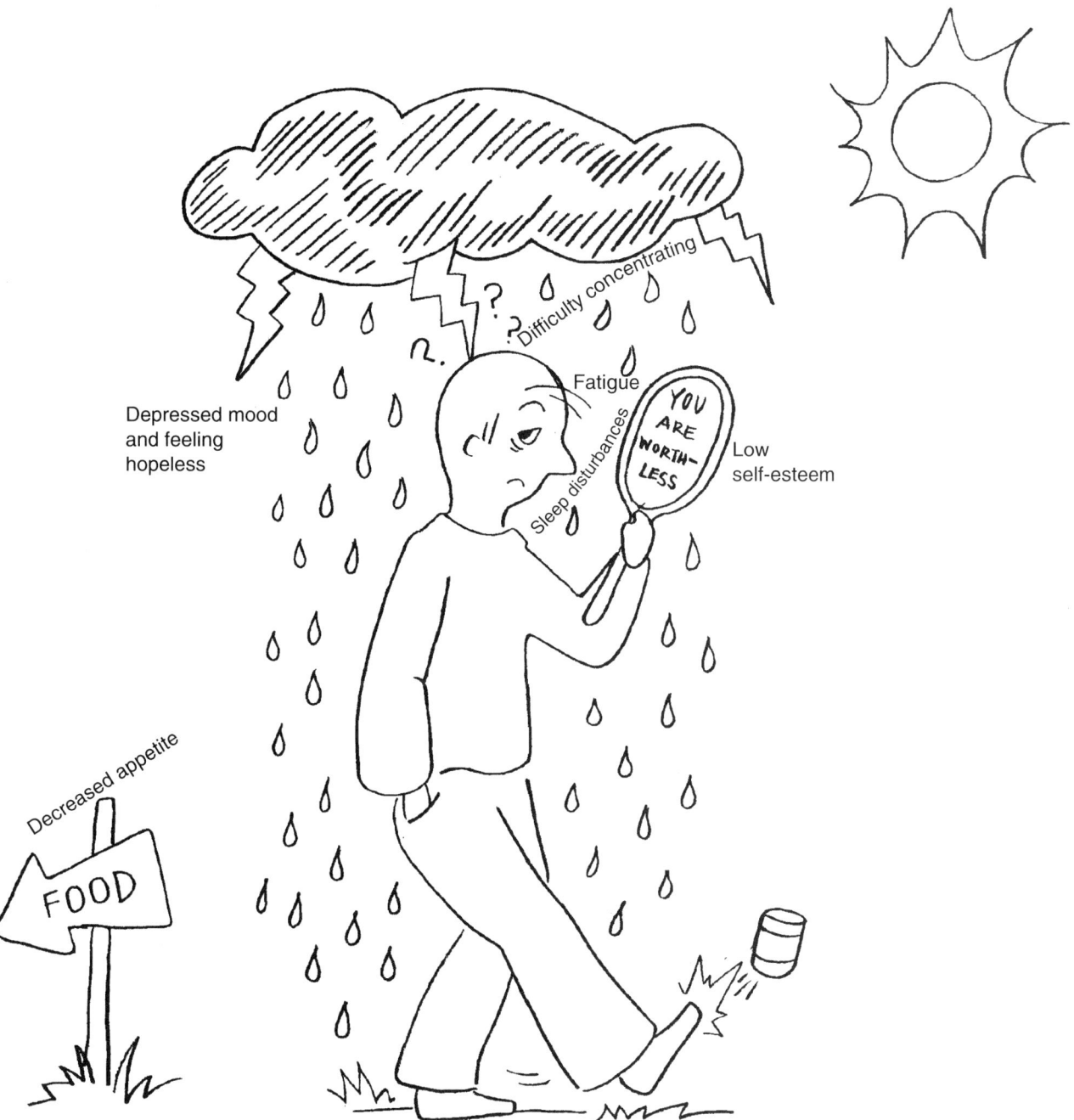

3. Mood Disorders

NOTES

BIPOLAR I AND BIPOLAR II (AS DEFINED BY DSM-IV-TR)

- Manic episode
    - During a one-week or longer period of elevated or irritable mood
    - During the episode, three or more of the following symptoms were present (four if mood was irritable):
        - Inflated self-esteem
        - Decreased need for sleep
        - More talkative
        - Flight of ideas (thoughts racing)
        - Distractible
        - Increase in goal-directed activity
        - Excessive participation in pleasurable activities that could have distressing outcomes (e.g., buying sprees, sexual indiscretions)
    - Episode causes social or occupational impairment, requires hospitalization, or psychotic features are present
- Mixed episode
    - Criteria are met for both manic and major depressive episode for at least one week
- Hypomanic episode
    - During a four-day period or longer, an elevated or irritable mood is present
    - During the episode, three or more of the following symptoms were present (four if mood was irritable):
        - Inflated self-esteem
        - Decreased need for sleep
        - More talkative
        - Flight of ideas (thoughts racing)
        - Distractible
        - Increase in goal-directed activity
        - Excessive participation in pleasurable activities that could have distressing outcomes (e.g., buying sprees, sexual indiscretions)
    - Episode not severe enough to cause social or occupational impairment as in a manic episode
- Bipolar I has six separate categories: single manic episode; most recent episode hypomanic; most recent episode manic; most recent episode mixed; most recent episode depressed; most recent episode unspecified
    - Each category meeting the criteria for the type of episode explained above and a history of at least one manic episode
- Bipolar II is categorized as having recurrent major depressive episodes with hypomanic episodes but never a manic or mixed episode
- Traditional treatment is lithium, but other choices include Tegretol and Depakote

Bipolar I and Bipolar II

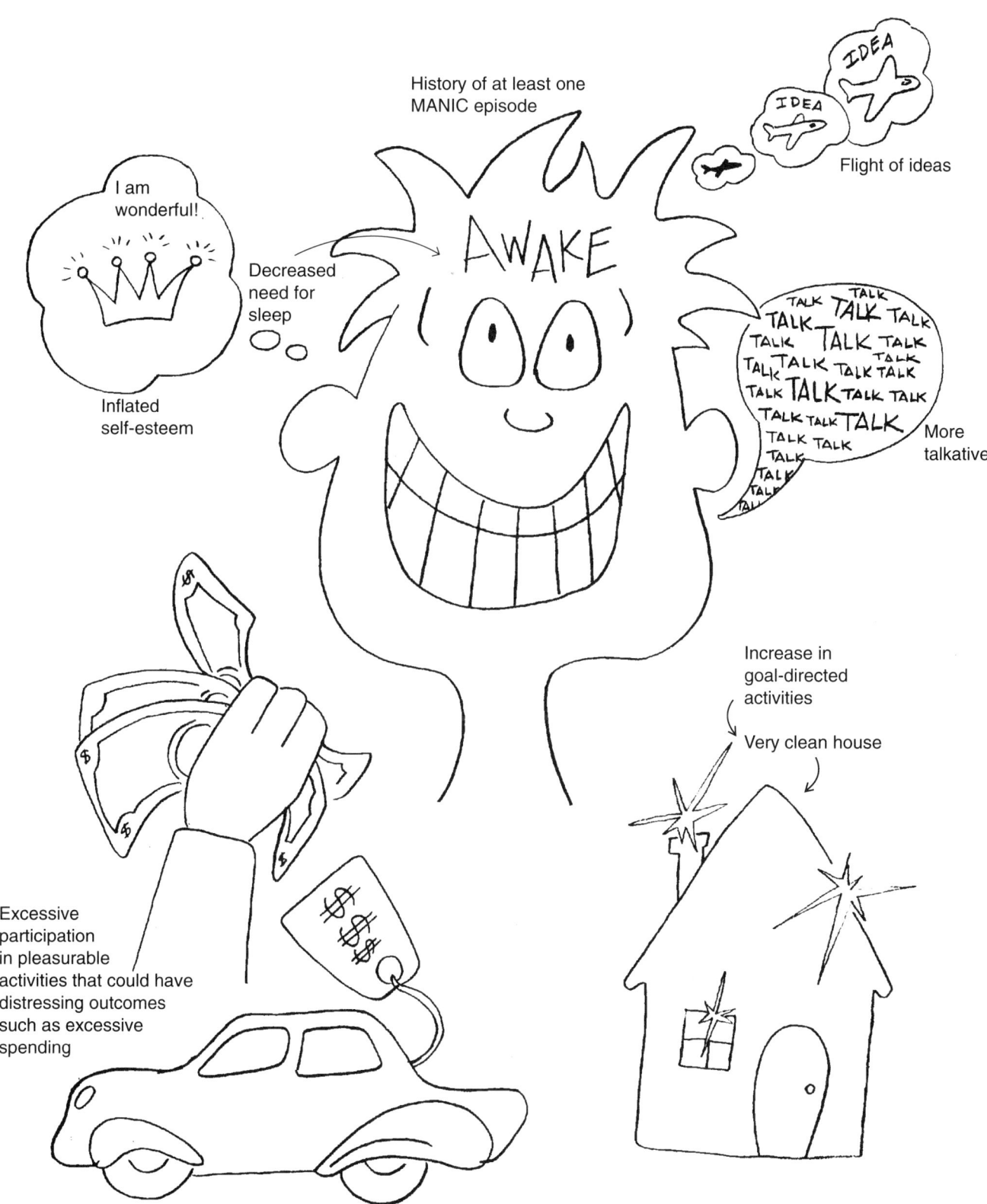

3. Mood Disorders

NOTES

CYCLOTHYMIC DISORDER (AS DEFINED BY DSM-IV-TR)

- During a two-year period, patient has multiple episodes of hypomania and multiple episodes of depressive symptoms that do not meet major depressive episode criteria
- During two-year period, person never went without symptoms for more than two months
- Episodes are not accounted for by other disorders, and there has never been a manic, mixed, or hypomanic episode

Cyclothymic Disorder

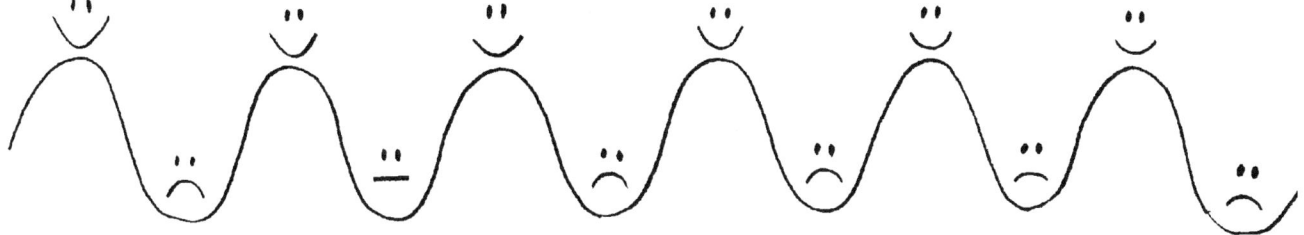

4. Personality Disorders

NOTES

PERSONALITY DISORDERS

- Coded on Axis II
- General diagnostic criteria include deviations of one's behavior from socially acceptable norms in two or more areas: cognition (interpretations of self and others), affectivity (emotional response), interpersonal functioning, and impulse control
- Pattern inflexible and occurs in many situations
- Causes distress and impairment of social functioning
- Pattern began in childhood or early adulthood

■ CLUSTER A PERSONALITY DISORDERS (DSM-IV-TR CRITERIA)

- **Paranoid**
  - Suspicious and distrustful of others and present in many contexts, and indicated by four (or more) of the following:
    - Suspects others are out to harm or deceive him or her
    - Preoccupied with unjustified doubts of loyalty of friends
    - Resists confiding in others for fear that the information will be used against him or her maliciously
    - Interprets benign remarks as harmful or threatening
    - Holds grudges
    - Misperception that individuals are attacking his or her character when it is not apparent to others; quick to counterattack
    - Recurrent unfounded suspicions about fidelity of spouse or sexual partner
- **Schizoid**
  - Pattern of social detachment and restricted emotional expression, and has four or more of the following:
    - Does not desire close relationships
    - Prefers solitude
    - No interest in sexual activities with another individual
    - Finds little pleasure in activities
    - Lacks close relationships other than family
    - Indifferent to praise or criticism
    - Flattened affectivity
- **Schizotypal**
  - Pattern of reduced capacity for close relationships, distorted perceptions, and eccentric behavior and appearance, and has five or more of the following:
    - Ideas of reference (impression that activities or remarks of others refer to one's self)
    - Odd beliefs or magical thinking (e.g., belief in telepathy, etc.)
    - Odd thought processes and speech
    - Suspicious ideation
    - Constricted or inappropriate affect
    - Eccentric or odd behavior and appearance
    - Lacks close relationships other than family

Cluster A Personality Disorders

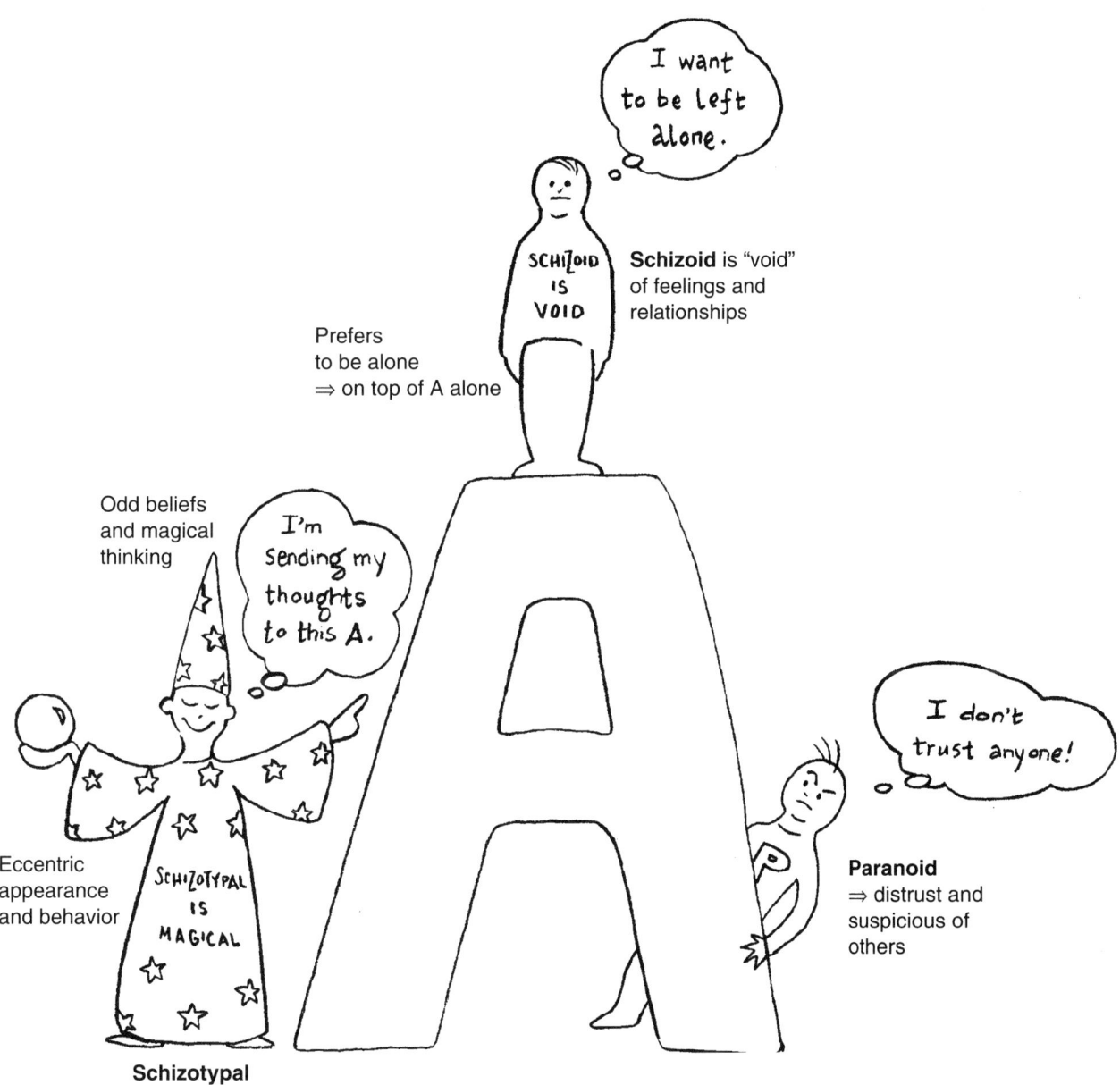

4. Personality Disorders

NOTES

■ CLUSTER B PERSONALITY DISORDERS (DSM-IV-TR CRITERIA)

- **Antisocial Personality Disorder**
    - Pattern of disregard for others since age of 15 years, with three or more of the following:
        - Does not conform to social norms regarding lawful behavior (repeatedly performs acts that are grounds for arrest)
        - Repeated lying
        - Impulsivity
        - Aggressiveness (repeated physical fights)
        - Disregard for others' safety
        - Consistent irresponsibility
        - Lack of remorse

      Individual must be 18 years or older, and there must be evidence of conduct disorder before the age of 15 years old.

- **Borderline Personality Disorder**
    - Pattern of instability of interpersonal relationships, self-image, and affects; impulsivity; and five or more of the following:
        - Frantic efforts to avoid abandonment
        - Unstable and intense interpersonal relationships
        - Unstable self-image
        - Impulsivity in areas that are potentially self-damaging (e.g., sex, spending, etc.)
        - Recurrent suicidal behavior or self-mutilating behavior
        - Affective instability
        - Chronic empty feeling
        - Difficulty controlling temper
        - Transient, stress-related paranoid ideation

- **Histrionic Personality Disorder**
    - Excessive emotionality and attention seeking, with five or more of the following:
        - Must be center of attention
        - Inappropriate sexually seductive or provocative behavior
        - Shallow emotions
        - Uses physical appearance to draw attention to self
        - Speech lacks detail
        - Self-dramatization
        - Suggestible
        - Believes relationships are more intimate than they actually are

- **Narcissistic Personality Disorder**
    - Pattern of grandiosity, need for admiration, and lack of empathy, with five or more of the following:
        - Grandiose sense of self-importance (e.g., exaggerates achievements, etc.)
        - Fantasies of success, power, brilliance, etc.
        - Believes he or she is special and can only mingle with important people
        - Requires excessive admiration
        - Sense of entitlement
        - Exploitative of others for self-gain
        - Lacks empathy
        - Envious of others
        - Arrogant or haughty attitudes

Cluster B Personality Disorders

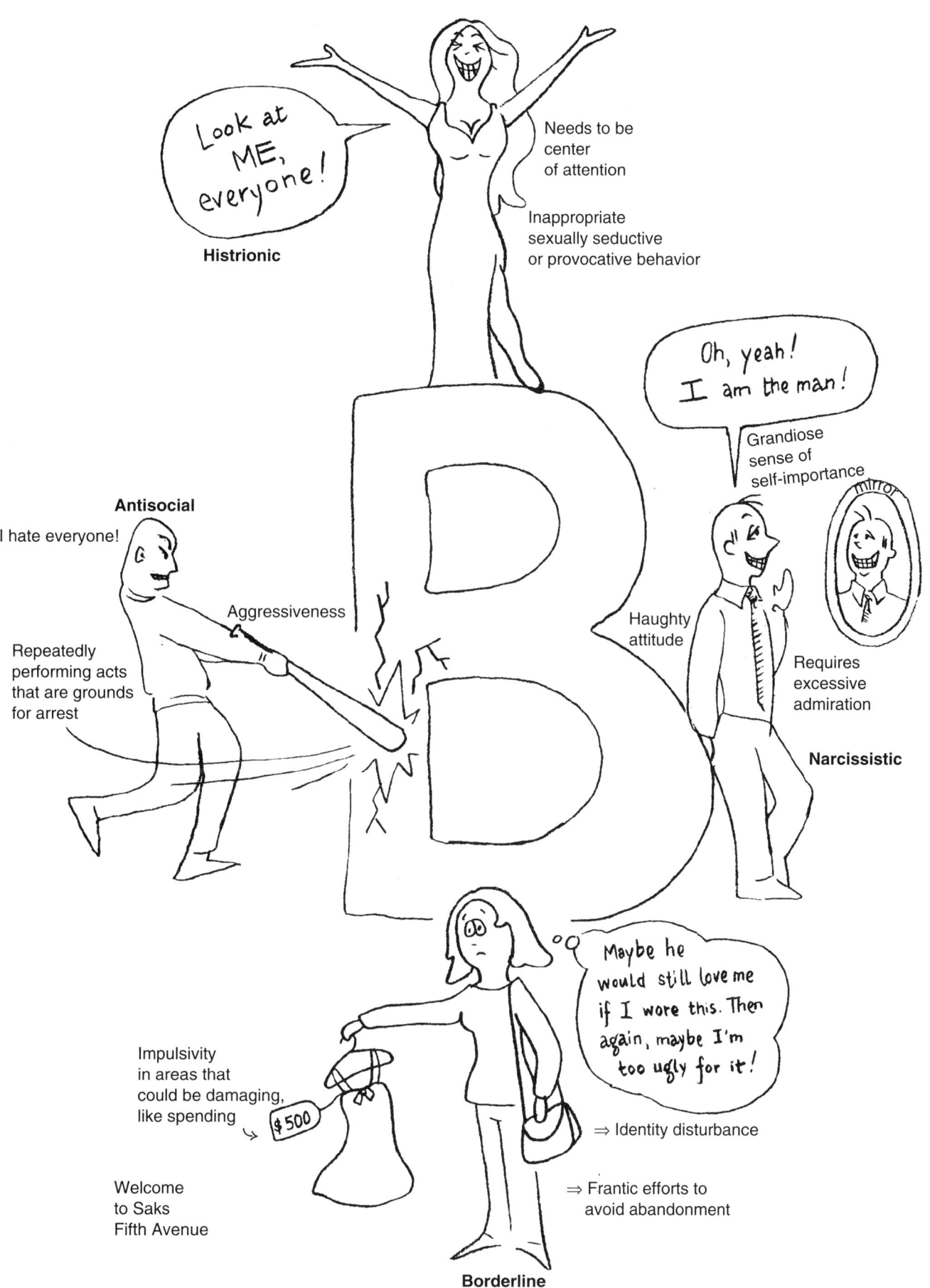

4. Personality Disorders

NOTES

■ CLUSTER C PERSONALITY DISORDERS (DSM-IV-TR CRITERIA)

- **Avoidant Personality Disorder**
    - Social inhibition, feels inadequate, hypersensitive to criticism, with four or more of the following:
        - Avoids occupational activities with a large proportion of interpersonal contact secondary to fear of criticism or rejection
        - Will only become involved with individuals if assured of positive outcome
        - Restraint within intimate relationships
        - Preoccupied about criticism in social situations
        - Inhibited in new relationships because of feelings of inadequacy
        - Views self as inferior or socially inept
        - Avoids new situations because of concerns they may be embarrassing
- **Dependent Personality Disorder**
    - Excessive need to be taken care of that leads to clingy behavior and fears of separation, with five or more of following:
        - Requires excessive advice to make everyday decisions
        - Needs others to assume responsibility
        - Difficulty expressing disagreement
        - Difficulty initiating projects (lack of self-confidence)
        - Goes to extreme lengths to obtain others' approval or nurturance
        - Feels helpless
        - Quickly moves to another relationship when one ends
        - Preoccupied with fears of being left alone
- **Obsessive-Compulsive Personality Disorder**
    - Obsession with orderliness and perfectionism; mental and interpersonal control; inflexible; with four or more of following:
        - Preoccupied with details and organization
        - Perfectionist
        - Workaholic; excludes leisure activities
        - Inflexible about morality and ethics
        - Cannot delegate tasks
        - Hoards money
        - Rigid and stubborn
        - Cannot discard worn-out items (even though they have no sentimental value)

Cluster C Personality Disorders

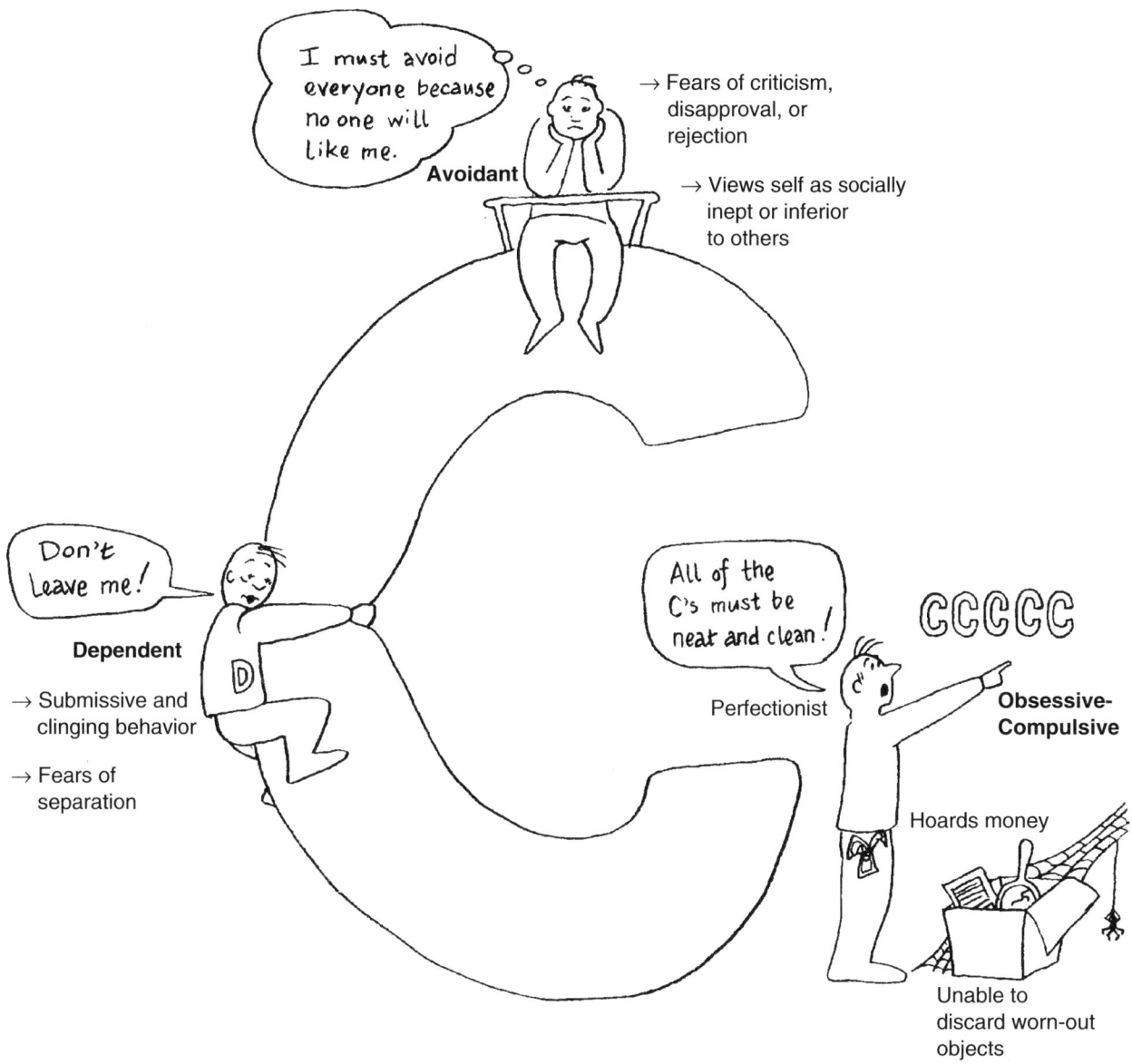

5. Anxiety Disorders

NOTES

GENERALIZED ANXIETY DISORDER

- According to DSM-IV-TR: Excessive anxiety and worry, occurring for at least six months, about several situations and/or activities
- It is difficult for individual to control the worry
- Individual must have at least three of six of the following associated symptoms:
  - Restlessness
  - Easily fatigued
  - Difficulty with concentration
  - Irritability
  - Muscle tension
  - Sleep disturbance
- Treatment
  - Pharmacologic: Antianxiety agents (benzodiazepines, buspirone, β-blockers) and antidepressants (especially selective serotonin reuptake inhibitors [SSRIs])
  - Psychological: Systemic desensitization, behavioral therapies (flooding), and support groups

Generalized Anxiety Disorder

27

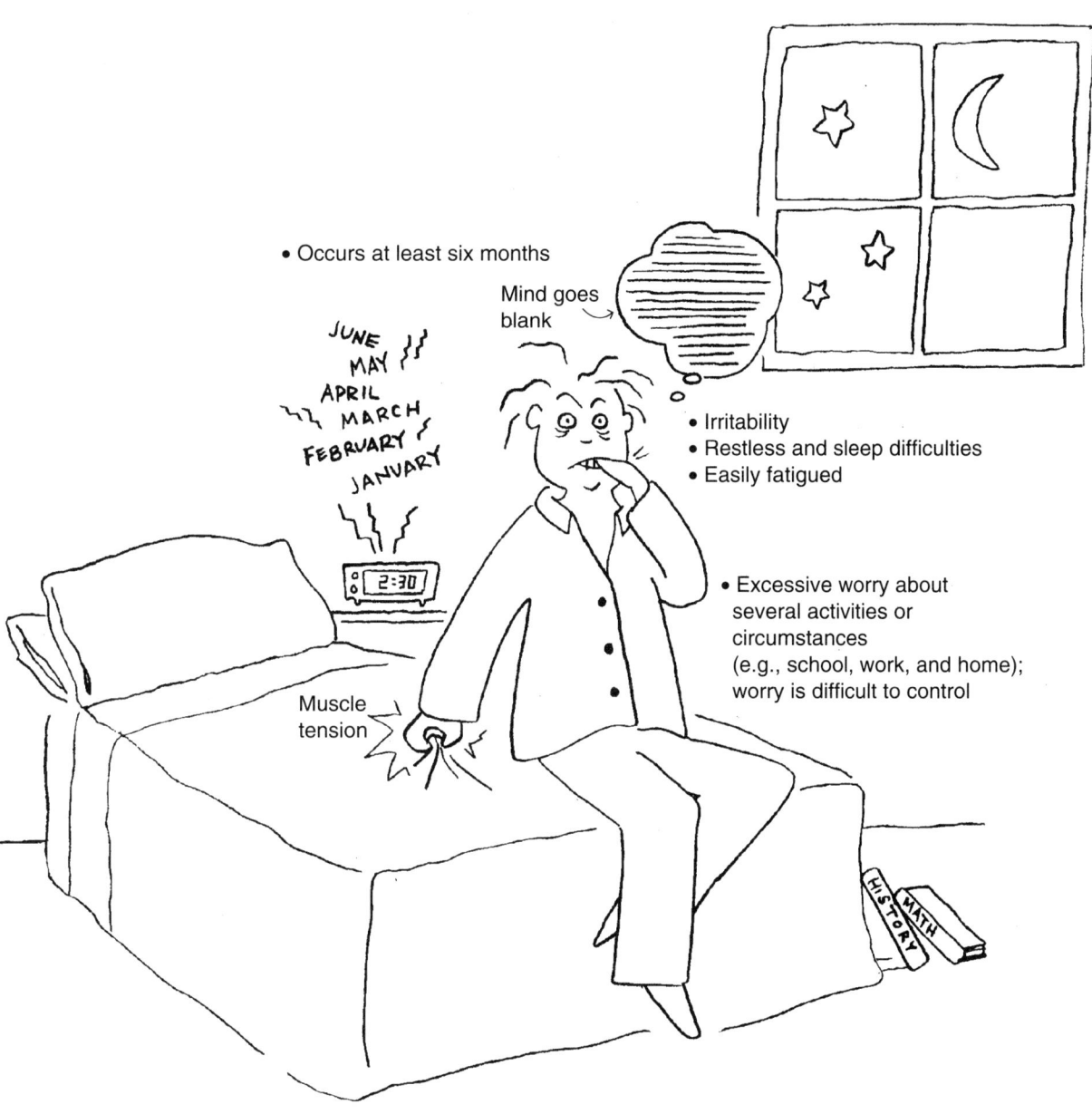

5. Anxiety Disorders

OBSESSIVE-COMPULSIVE DISORDER (OCD)

- Obsessions
  - Recurrent thoughts or images that cause marked anxiety
  - Thoughts and anxiety beyond normal worries of daily life
  - Person attempts to stop thoughts because he or she realizes that thoughts are initiated in own mind (patient has insight into illness)
- Compulsions
  - Repetitive behaviors that the patient feels driven to complete to prevent dreaded happenings or to relieve stress
- Obsessions or compulsions consume more than an hour per day
- Treatment:
  - Pharmacologic: Antianxiety agents (benzodiazepines, buspirone, β-blockers) and antidepressants (especially selective serotonin reuptake inhibitors [SSRIs] like fluoxetine)
  - Psychological: Systemic desensitization, behavioral therapies (flooding), and support groups

Obsessive-Compulsive Disorder (OCD)

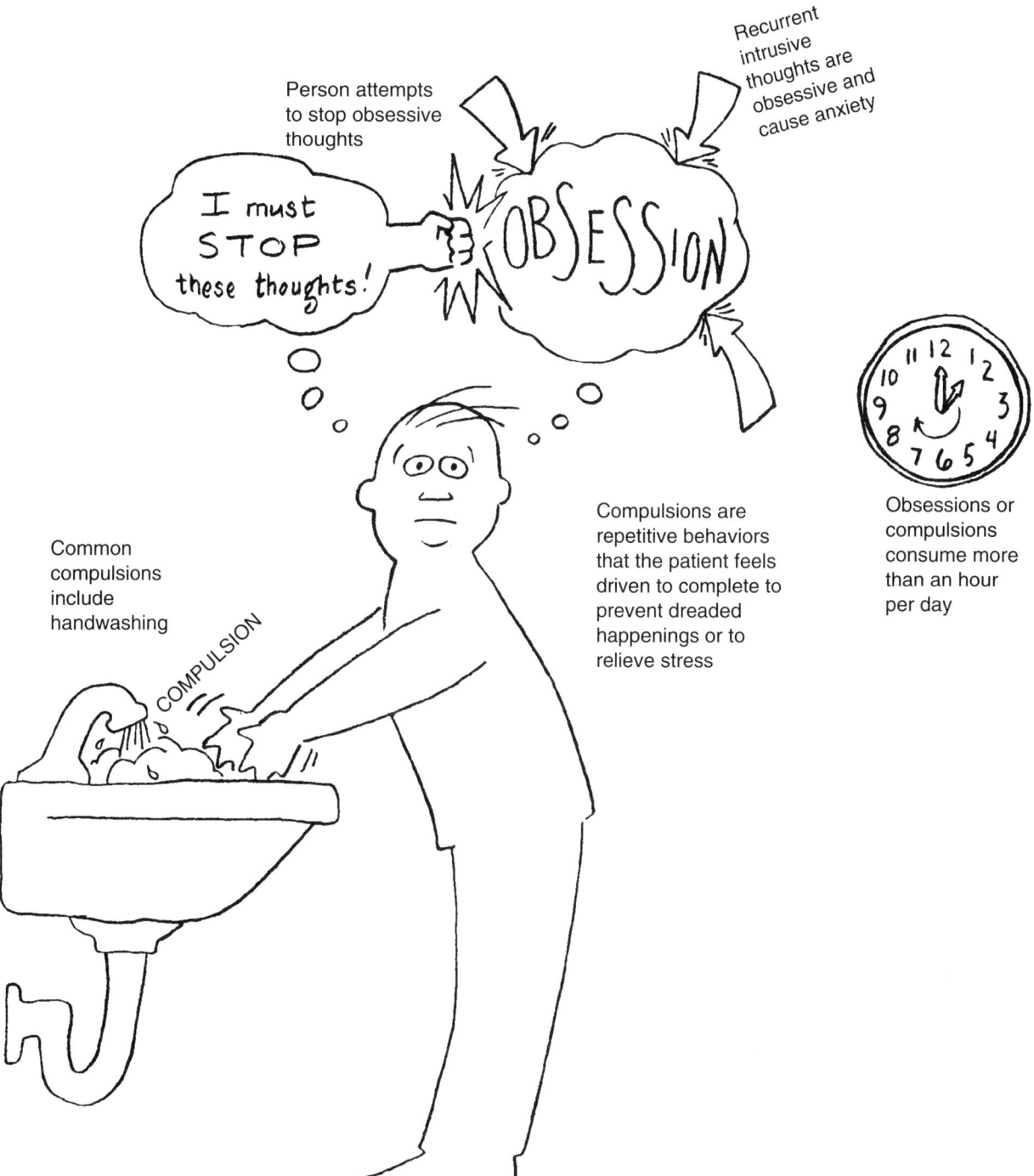

5. Anxiety Disorders

NOTES

POST-TRAUMATIC STRESS DISORDER

- Person exposed to a traumatic event in which following occurred (DSM-IV-TR):
  - Person experienced or witnessed life-threatening event
  - Person's response involved intense fear
- Event continually relived in following manner:
  - Recurrent, intrusive, and distressing thoughts or images
  - Recurrent nightmares
  - Feels as if reliving experience often
  - Psychological distress and physiologic response to stimuli that resembles aspect of event or exaggerated startle response
- Avoidance of stimuli, conversation, thoughts, or feelings associated with traumatic event
- Hypervigilance or exaggerated startle response
- Symptoms have occurred for longer than one month

Post-Traumatic Stress Disorder

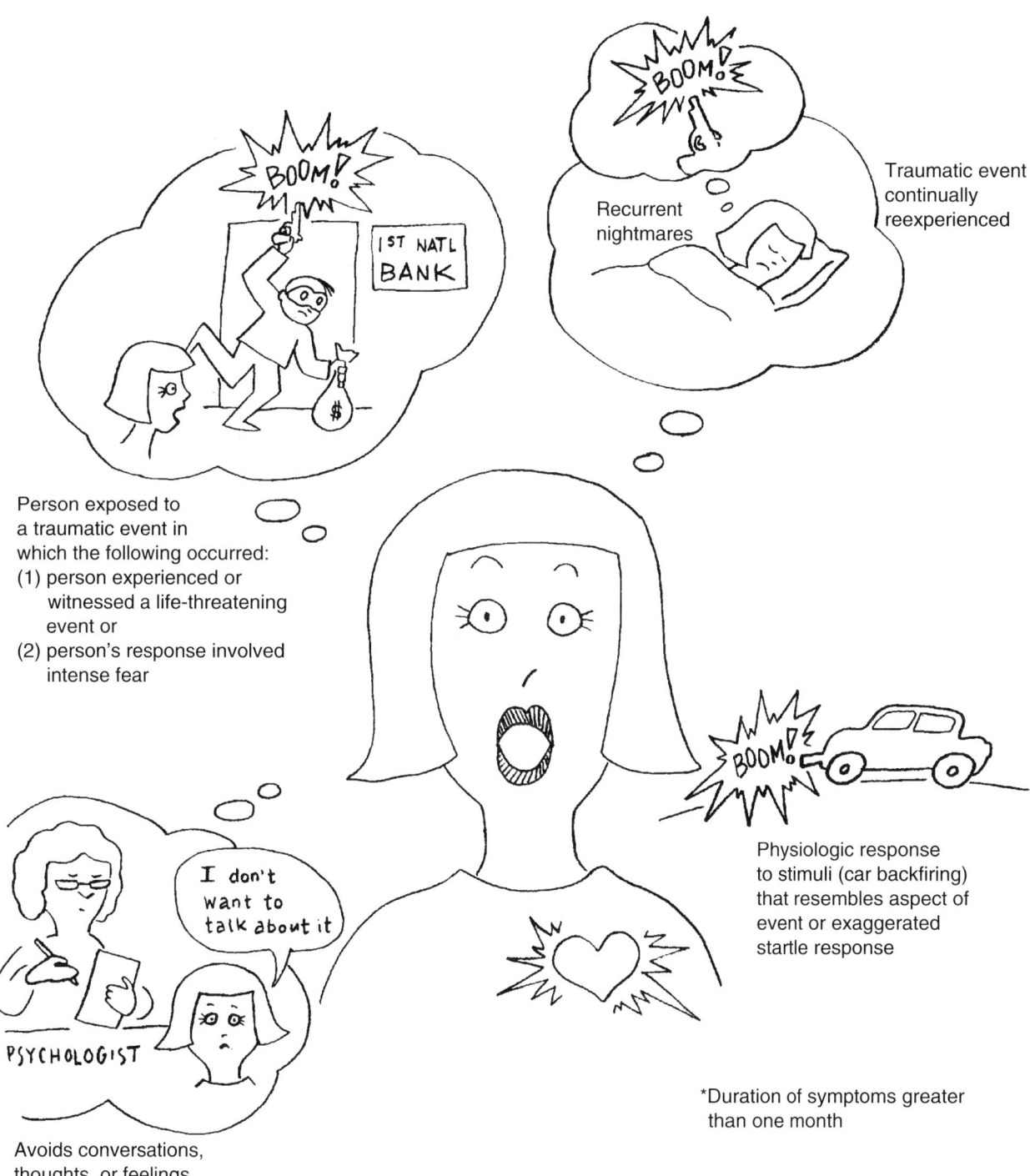

5. Anxiety Disorders

NOTES

PANIC DISORDER

- Both of the following must occur according to DSM-IV-TR:
  - Recurrent panic attacks
  - One panic attack, at least, followed by one or more of these symptoms for one month:
    - Worrying about further attacks
    - Concerns for health and physical implications of attacks (e.g., heart attack)
    - Change in behavior secondary to attacks
- Can occur with or without agoraphobia (see Phobia chapter for more information regarding agoraphobia)

Panic Disorder

(can occur with or without agoraphobia*)

MARCH

sunday	monday	tuesday	wednesday	thursday	friday	saturday
PANIC ATTACK — 1	What if I have another? — 2	Maybe I am going CRAZY! — 3	4	5	6	What if I have a heart attack after one? — 7
8	I can't go anywhere because I might have one! — 9	10	11	I know I'm going to have one any day now! — 12	13	14
15	16	17	18	19	20	21
22	23	24	25	26	27	28
29	30	31				

Recurrent panic attacks with at least one of the panic attacks followed by concerns for one month

*See illustration regarding agoraphobia in Phobia chapter

6. Somatoform Disorders, Factitious Disorders, and Malingering

SOMATOFORM DISORDERS: SOMATIZATION

- Long, chronic history of multiple complaints
  - "I'm always sick!"
- Criteria include:
  - Four pain symptoms related to four different locations or functions (e.g., headache, abdominal pain)
    ⇒ four fingers
  - Two gastrointestinal (GI) symptoms (e.g., nausea, constipation)
  - One pseudoneurologic symptom (e.g., seizure, paralysis)
  - One sexual symptom (e.g., heavy or absent menstrual cycles)
- Symptoms not caused by medical condition
- Patient truly believes symptoms are real
- Symptoms not produced intentionally
- Most common in females
- Onset occurs before 30 years of age
- Often seen by several physicians and receives multiple treatments for symptoms
- Illnesses with multiple symptoms, such as systemic lupus erythematosus (SLE), multiple sclerosis, and HIV infection, must be excluded

Somatization Disorder

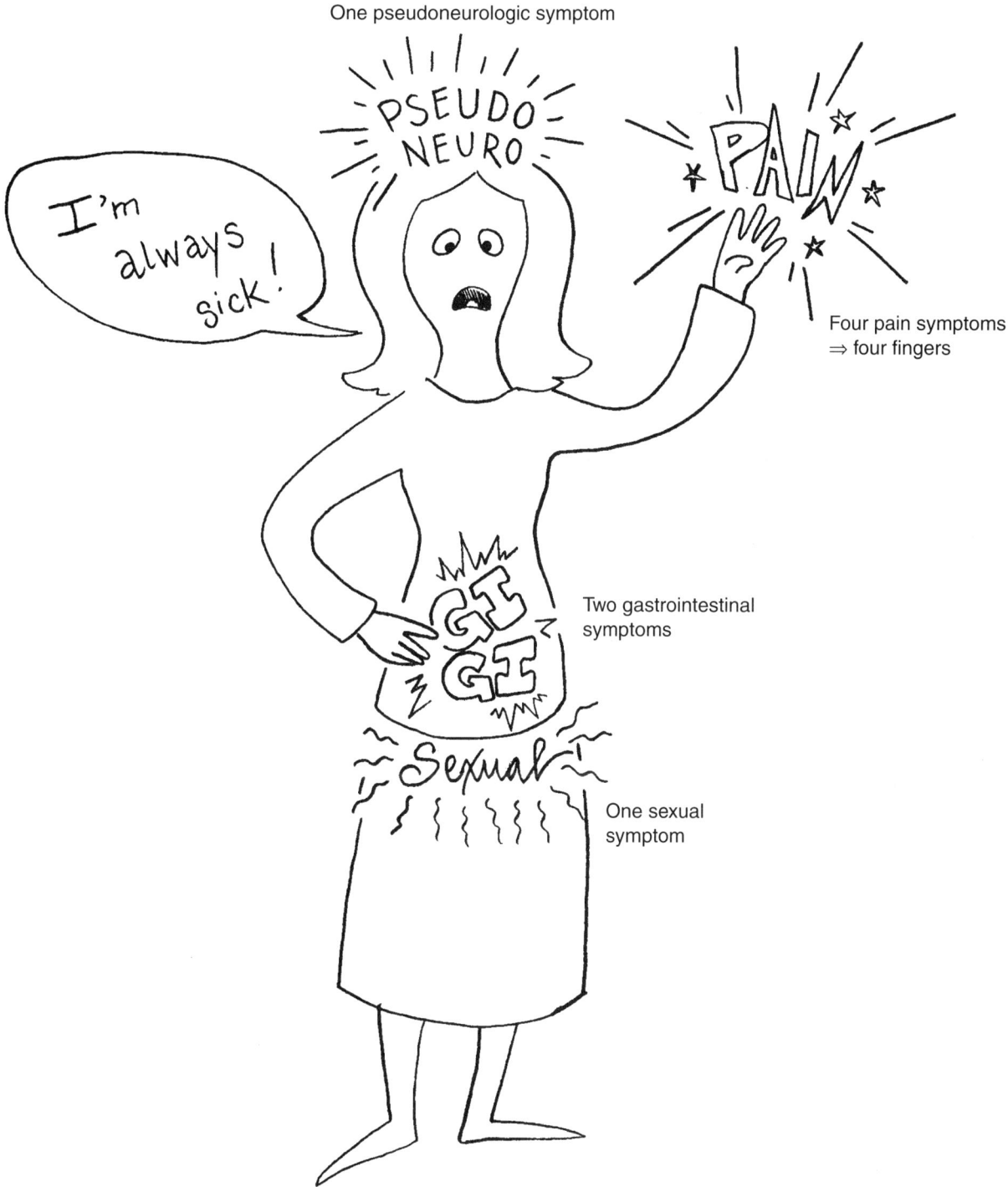

- Long, chronic history of multiple complaints
- Not caused by medical condition
- Patient truly believes symptoms are real
- Symptoms not produced willfully
- Most common in females
- Onset occurs before 30 years of age

6. Somatoform Disorders, Factitious Disorders, and Malingering

NOTES

SOMATOFORM DISORDERS: CONVERSION DISORDER

- Sudden loss of motor or sensory function
  - Common symptoms of motor loss include paralysis and seizures
    ⇒ paralysis = wheelchair
  - Common symptoms of sensory loss include vision loss, hearing loss, and numbness
    ⇒ vision loss = "Now I can't see!"
    ⇒ numbness = hand tingling
- Deficits are inconsistent with anatomic distribution
- Neurologic exam is often normal
- Symptoms not caused by a medical condition
- Often triggered by stress
  ⇒ STRESS running into wheelchair
- Patients often seem unconcerned about loss of function; termed "La Belle Indifference"
  ⇒ La Belle = the bell
- Treatment includes anxiolytics and relaxation techniques

Conversion Disorder

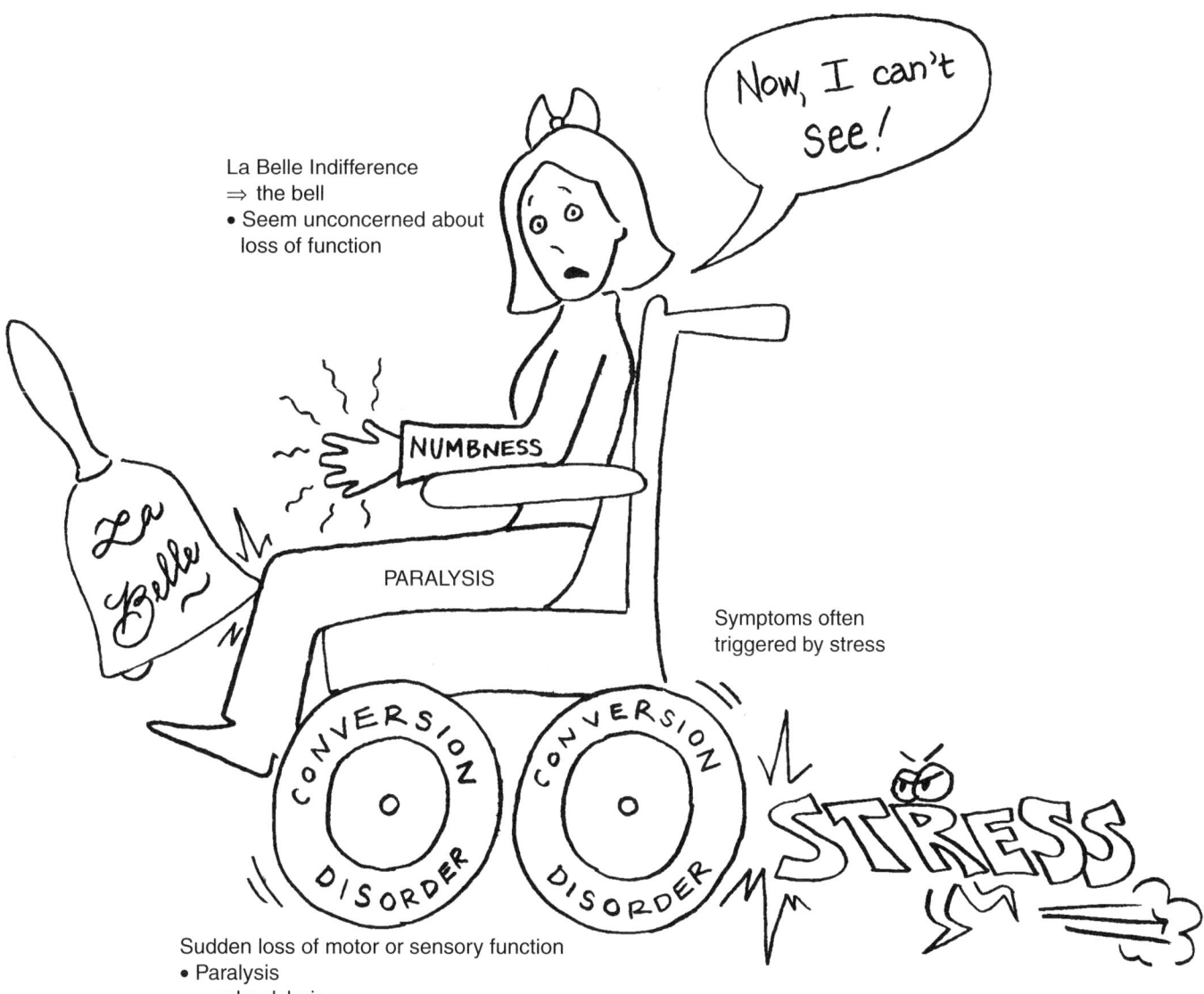

6. Somatoform Disorders, Factitious Disorders, and Malingering

SOMATOFORM DISORDERS: HYPOCHONDRIASIS

- Concerned with having a serious illness from misunderstanding normal bodily functions
    ⇒ "No, I know I have cancer!"
- Patient is still concerned despite normal medical evaluation
    ⇒ "Sir, that is a normal bodily function."
- Seen by many doctors, known as "doctor shopping"
    ⇒ "All of these doctors are wrong!"
- Occurs over at least a six-month period
    ⇒ six-month calendar

Hypochondriasis

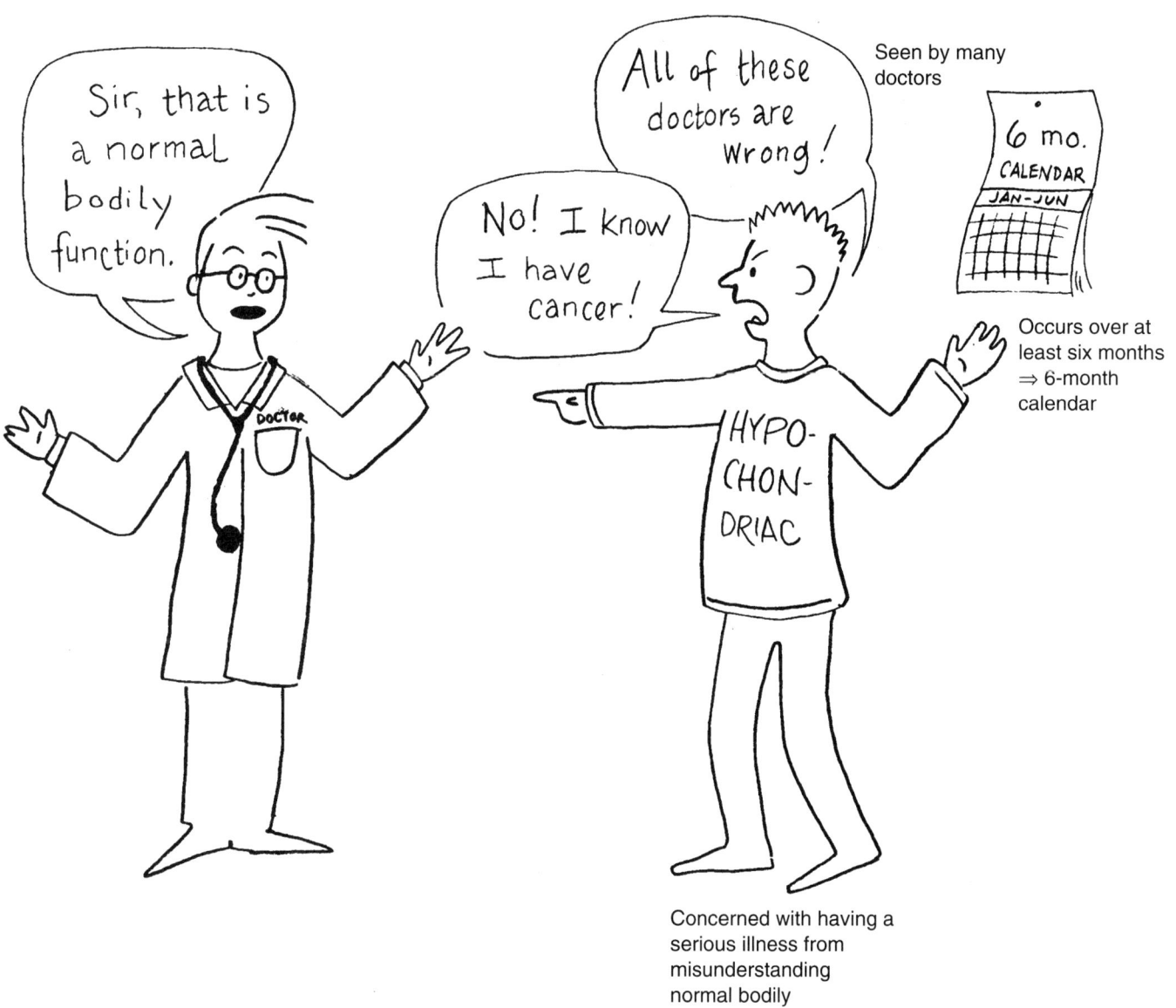

6. Somatoform Disorders, Factitious Disorders, and Malingering

SOMATOFORM DISORDERS: BODY DYSMORPHIC DISORDER

- Excessive concern with an imagined physical defect
  ⇒ "My nose is too big!" even though nose is normal size
- Imagined defect usually involves the face, head, hair, or body shape
- Preoccupation leads to functional impairment
  ⇒ "I can't go out!"
- Onset occurs in the teenage years
- Occurs in men and women with the same frequency
- Multiple visits with plastic surgeons common

Body Dysmorphic Disorder

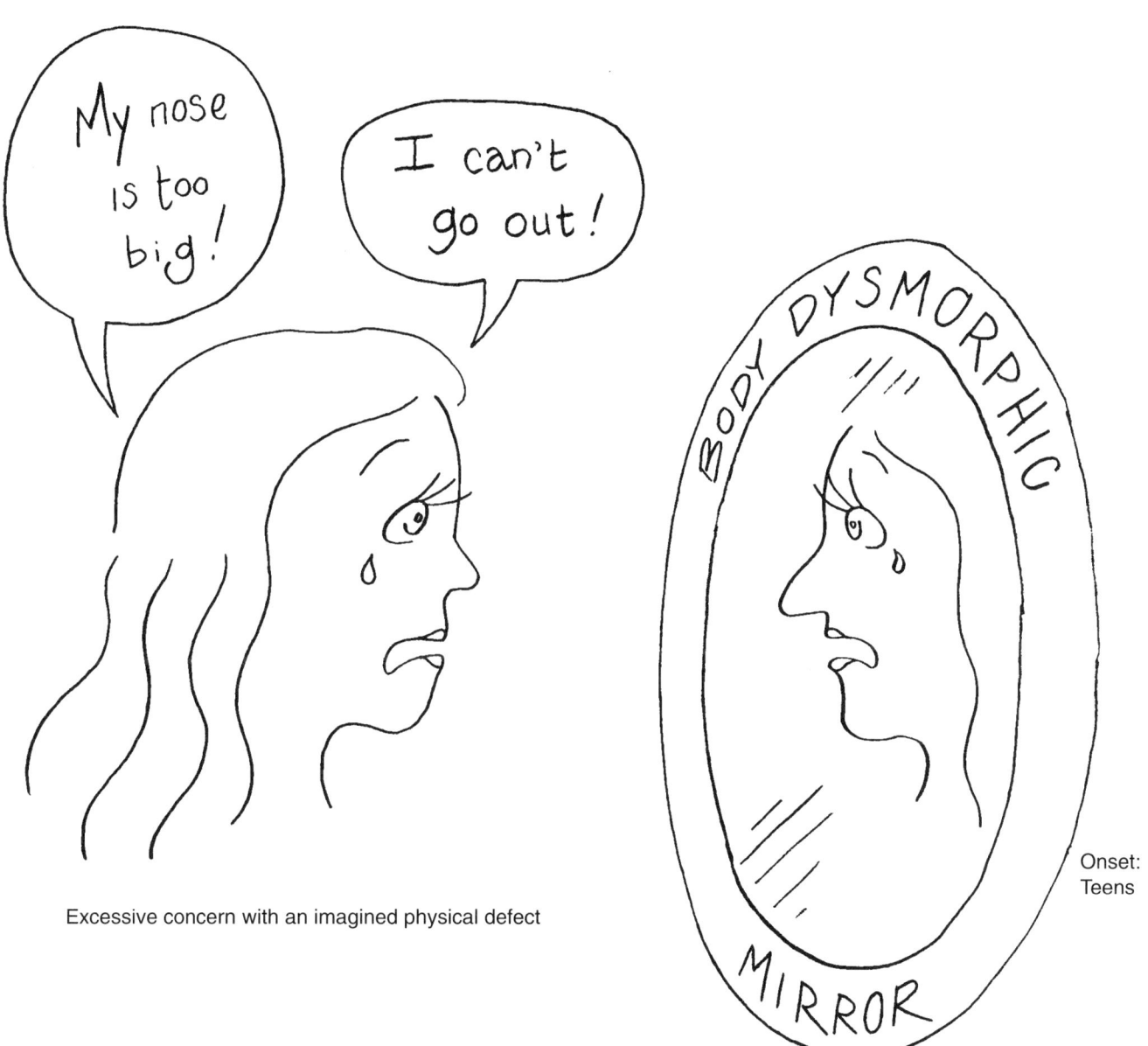

Excessive concern with an imagined physical defect

Onset: Teens

6. Somatoform Disorders, Factitious Disorders, and Malingering

SOMATOFORM DISORDERS: PAIN DISORDER

⇒ pain = bandage
- Pain complaints not fully explained by medical cause
- Severity is exaggerated
    ⇒ "My pain is severe!"
- May occur with a medical condition, but severity of pain not adequately explained
- Pain medication dependence may occur
    ⇒ pain pills
- Onset occurs at 30 to 40 years of age
- Treatment includes selective serotonin reuptake inhibitors (SSRIs)

Pain Disorder

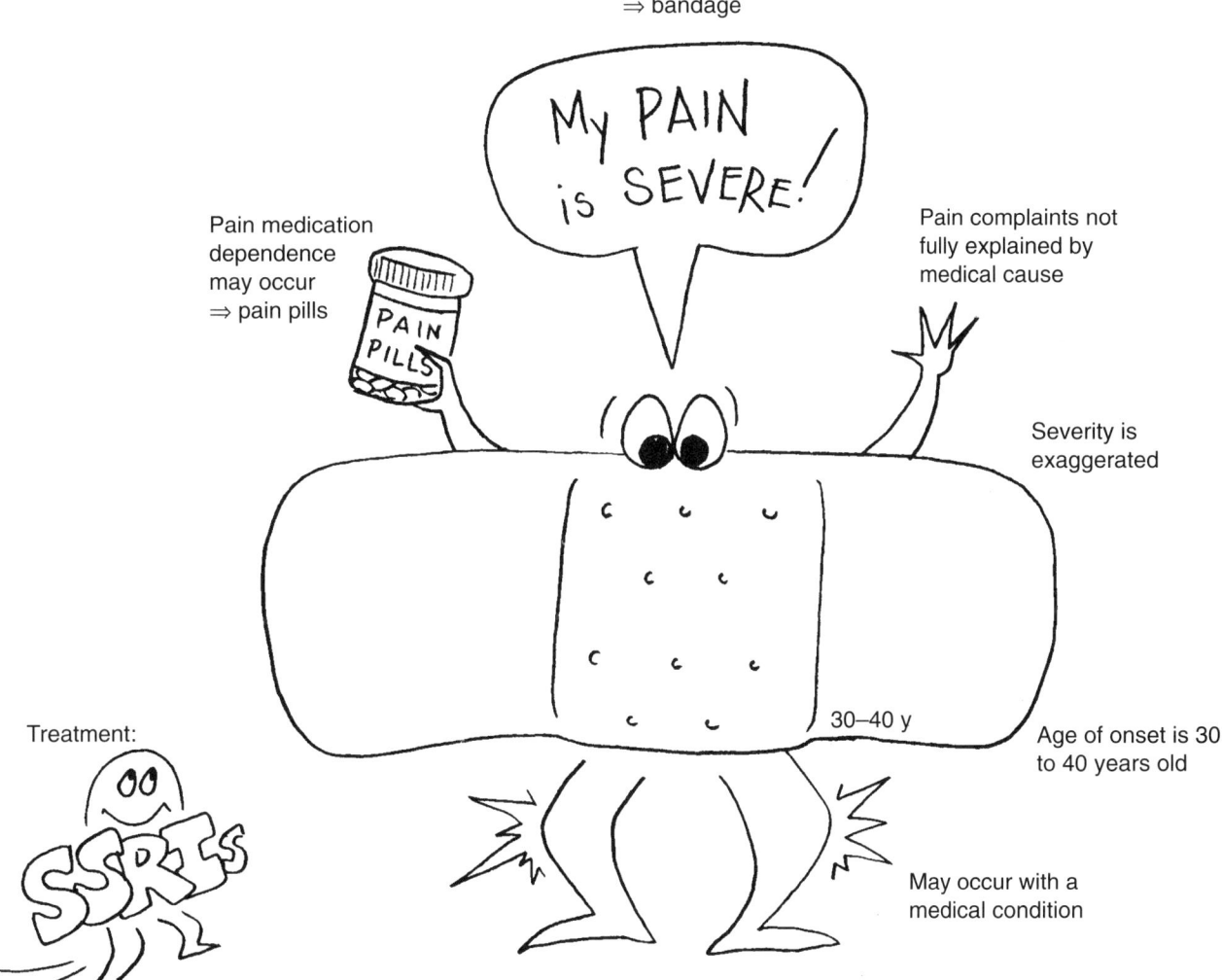

6. Somatoform Disorders, Factitious Disorders, and Malingering

FACTITIOUS DISORDER

- Patients with factitious disorder intentionally produce or fake symptoms of a mental or physical illness to gain medical attention
    - ⇒ medical attention = I ♥ Doctors on shirt
    - ⇒ intentionally produce symptoms = "I *know* I fake my symptoms!"
- Symptoms often faked include:
    - Seizures
        - ⇒ lightning bolts on head
    - Fever (patients may heat thermometer or skin)
        - ⇒ thermometer
    - Abdominal pain
        - ⇒ rubbing belly
- Symptoms produced include skin lesions and effects of medication use (e.g., insulin use leading to hypoglycemia)
- Factitious disorder involving mainly physical symptoms is also known as Munchausen's syndrome
- Factitious disorder by proxy (Munchausen's syndrome by proxy) involves an adult who fakes or induces an illness in a child to receive medical attention
    - ⇒ Munchausen's by proxy = baby in crib
- Patients often receive unnecessary medicines and multiple medical procedures
- Patients often have worked in the medical field
    - ⇒ stethoscope and nurse's hat
- Patients with somatoform disorders truly believe symptoms are real, in contrast to patients with factitious disorder, who know they produce or fake symptoms

Factitious Disorder

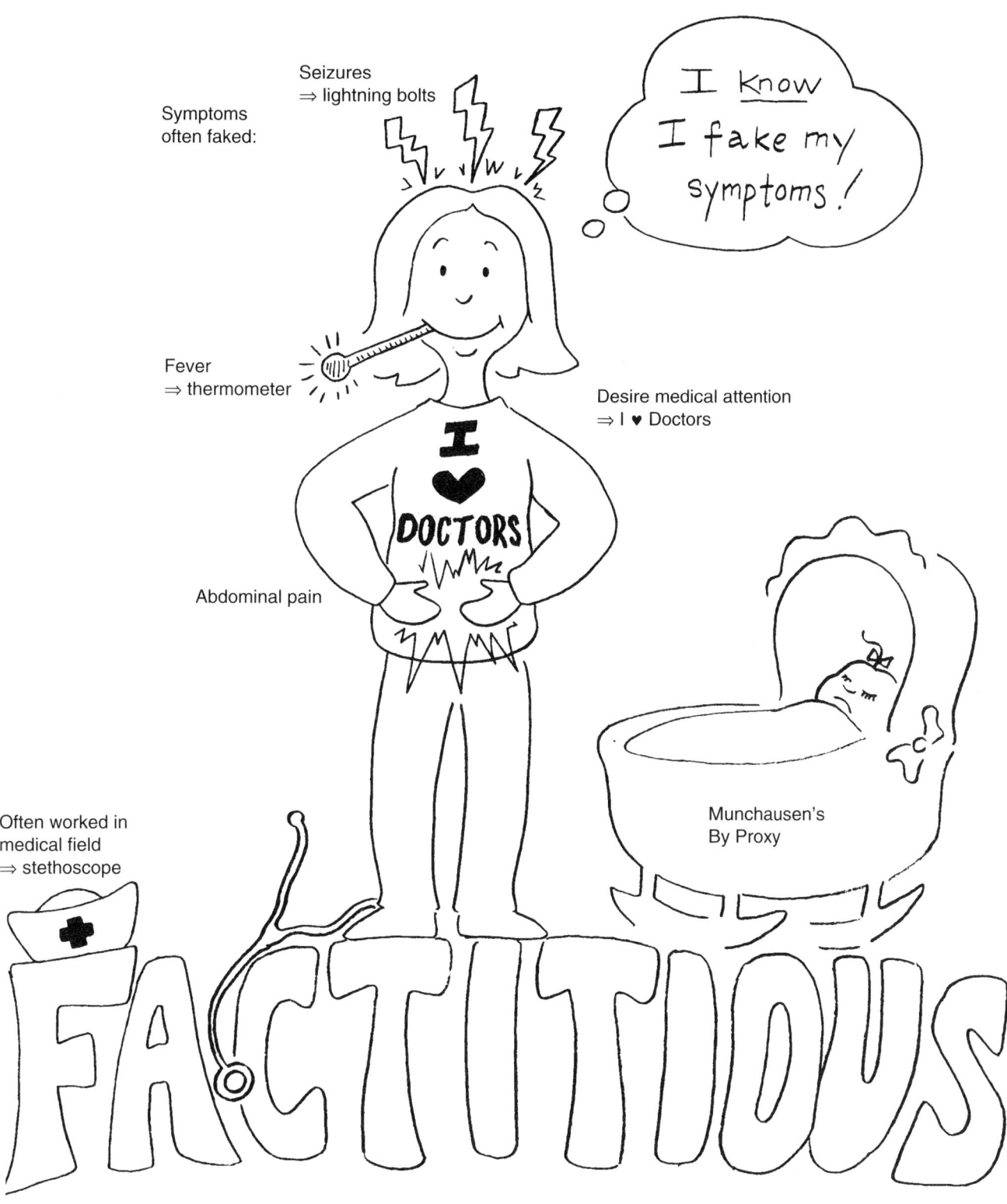

6. Somatoform Disorders, Factitious Disorders, and Malingering

NOTES

MALINGERING

- Malingering involves lying about symptoms of a mental or physical illness for financial or other gain, such as avoiding work or military service
    - ⇒ financial gain = bag of money
    - ⇒ avoiding work = I don't have to work 'cause I'm "sick"!
- Malingering patients avoid medical treatment, and symptoms often improve after obtaining gain

Malingering

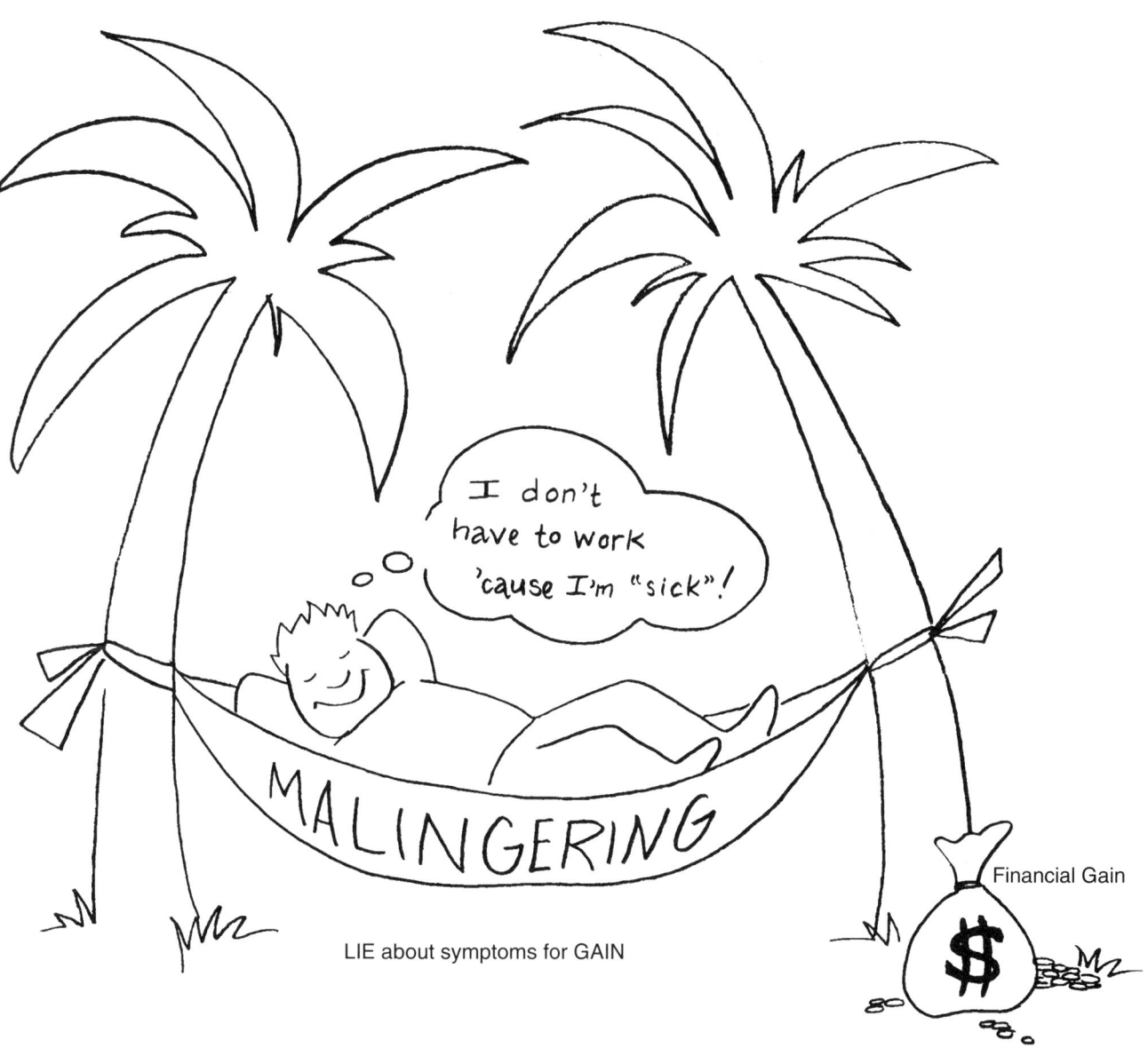

7. Substance Abuse

NOTES

ALCOHOL ABUSE (AS DEFINED BY DSM-IV-TR, THESE CRITERIA CAN ALSO BE USED TO DIAGNOSE ABUSE OF OTHER SUBSTANCES)

- During a 12-month period, one of the following must have occurred secondary to use of alcohol or any other substance:
  - Recurrent impairment in fulfillment of obligations at work, home, or school
  - Repeatedly putting one's self and others in harm's way secondary to alcohol use (e.g., driving while intoxicated)
  - Recurrent legal problems related to alcohol use (e.g., disorderly conduct, etc.)
  - Continued use of alcohol even after social, occupational, or personal consequences have taken place (e.g., spousal disruption secondary to alcohol intake)

ALCOHOL DEPENDENCE (AS DEFINED BY DSM-IV-TR, THESE CRITERIA CAN ALSO BE USED TO DIAGNOSE OTHER SUBSTANCE DEPENDENCE)

- Pattern of alcohol use leading to social, personal, or occupational impairment, as exemplified by three or more of the following having occurred in a 12-month period:
  - Tolerance (need for increased substance amounts in order to attain same effect as previously done with smaller amount or decreased effect over time when taking the same amount of the substance)
  - Withdrawal (achieves withdrawal syndrome of particular substance when not taken or need to take same substance or other substance to avoid withdrawal effects)
  - Increasing use of substance than previously intended
  - Repeated failures to stop use or decrease use of substance
  - Large amount of time devoted to substance either to attain it, use it, or recover from its effects
  - Decreased involvement in personal, occupational, and recreational activities secondary to substance use
  - Continued substance use even though individual knows substance makes physical or psychological problems worse
- Dependence specified as either with or without physiologic dependence (depending on evidence of tolerance or withdrawal)

Alcohol Abuse and Dependence

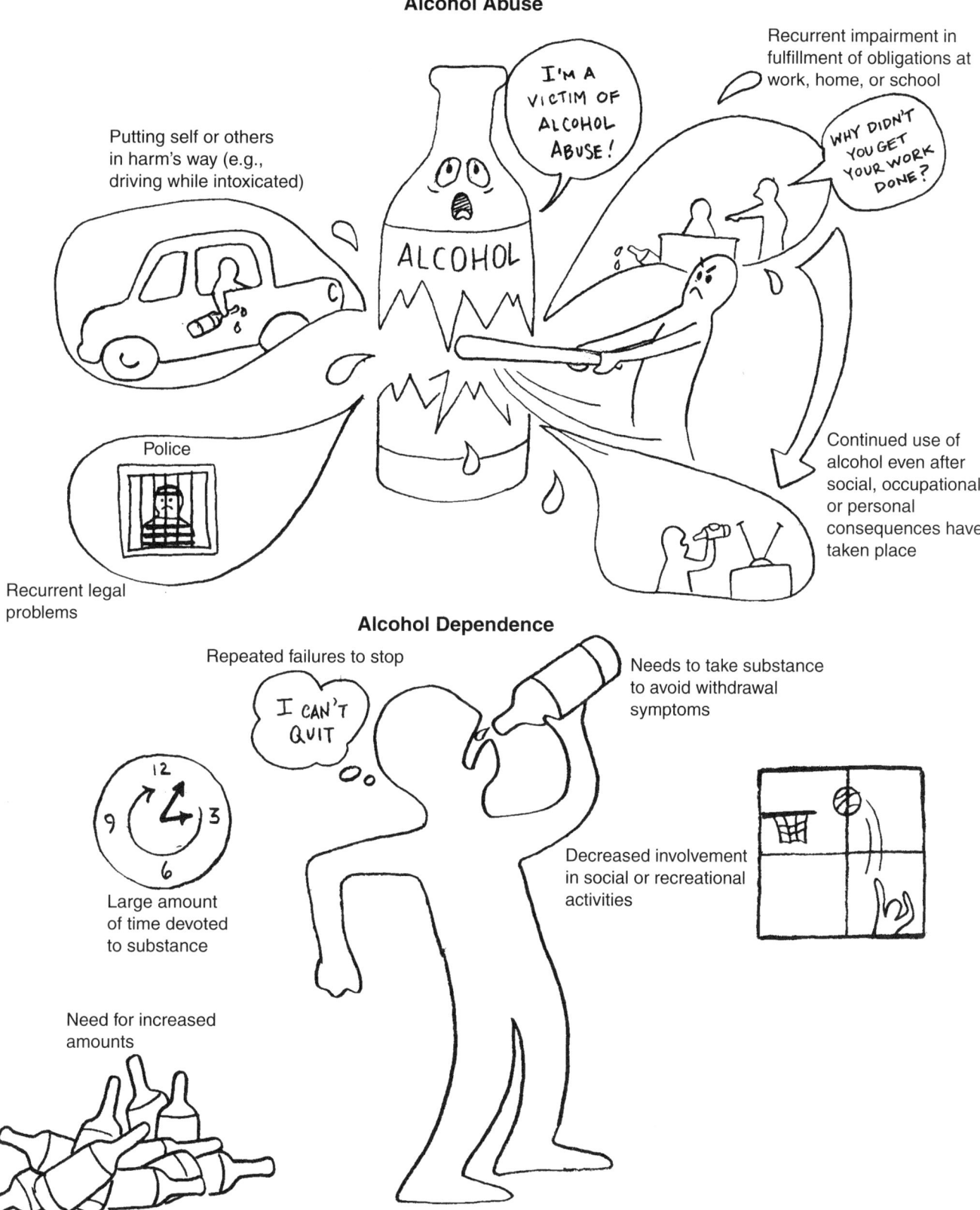

7. Substance Abuse

ALCOHOL INTOXICATION (AS DEFINED BY DSM-IV-TR)

- Recent alcohol intake
- After alcohol intake, substantial change in behavior occurs (e.g., increased aggressive or other inappropriate behaviors)
- After alcohol ingestion, one or more of the following occurs:
  - Slurred speech
  - Incoordination
  - Unsteady gait
  - Nystagmus
  - Memory impairment
  - Stupor or coma

ALCOHOL WITHDRAWAL (AS DEFINED BY DSM-IV-TR)

- Recent decrease in alcohol consumption that was previously quite heavy
- After cessation of alcohol intake, two or more of the following occur:
  - Autonomic hyperactivity
  - Increased hand tremor
  - Insomnia
  - Nausea/vomiting
  - Transient hallucinations
  - Psychomotor agitation
  - Anxiety
  - Grand mal seizures
- Symptoms cause significant social or occupational impairment

■ MISCELLANEOUS

- Chronic alcohol use associated with alcohol dementia
- Fetal alcohol syndrome occurs when mothers ingest large amounts of alcohol during pregnancy and include the following:
  - Microcephaly
  - Small for gestational age
  - Palpebral fissures
  - Epicanthal folds
  - Maxillary hypoplasia
  - Micrognathis
  - Thin vermilion of upper lip
  - Cleft palate
  - Irritability
  - Learning disorders
- Alcohol reacts with several receptors in the central nervous system (CNS), including facilitating gamma-aminobutyric acid (GABA)-induced inhibition; alcohol is also inhibitory to the glutamate (CNS excitatory neurotransmitter) receptor, thus causing sedation
- Treatment: Supportive and maintaining physiologic homeostasis
  - Patients in alcohol withdrawal syndrome may need pharmacologic intervention including benzodiazepines
  - Alcoholics with poor nutrition will need thiamine administration (before glucose administration) to prevent Wernicke-Korsakoff syndrome
  - Disulfiram is an irreversible inhibitor of acetaldehyde dehydrogenase, causing tachycardia, skin flushing, nausea, vomiting, and diaphoresis after alcohol consumption

Alcohol Intoxication

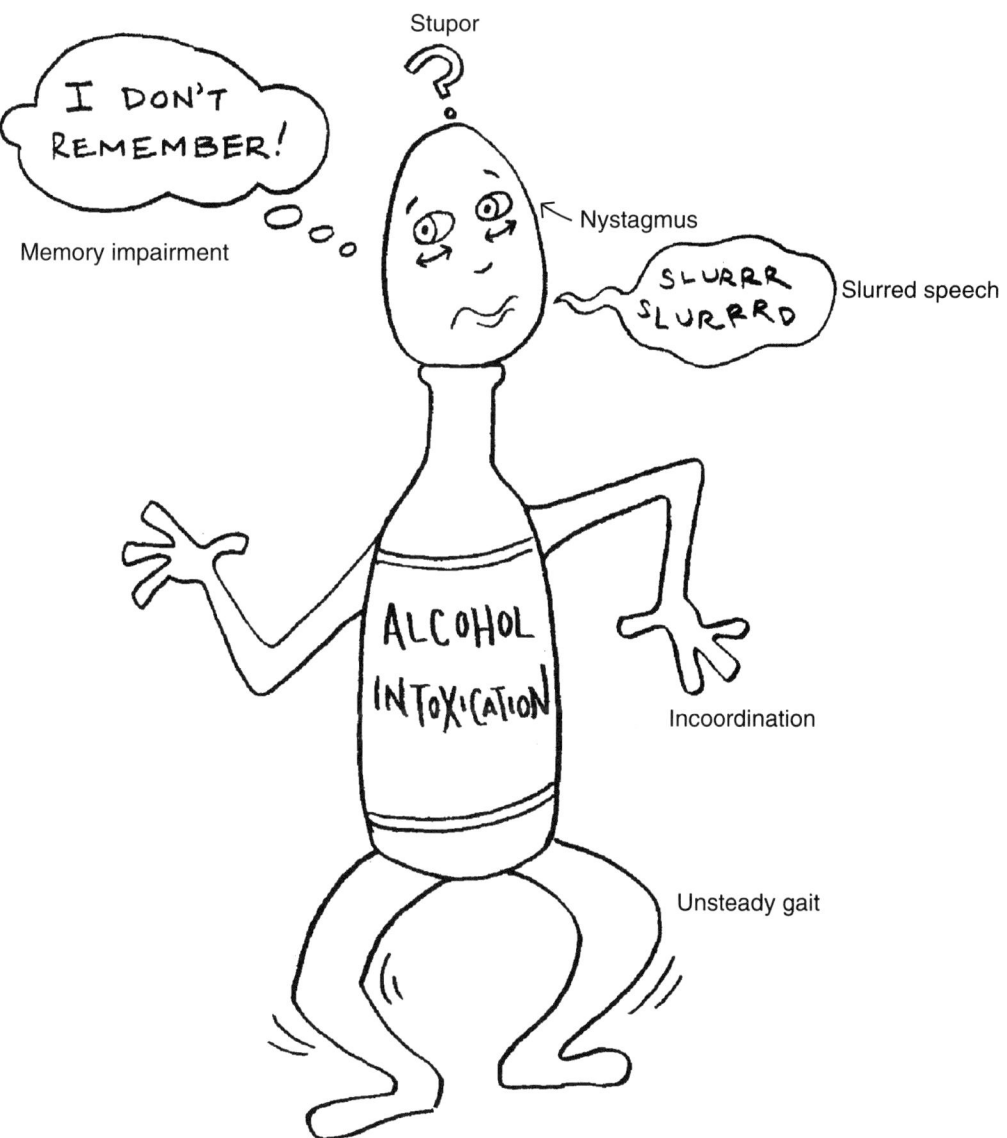

7. Substance Abuse

NOTES

AMPHETAMINE INTOXICATION (ACCORDING TO DSM-IV-TR CRITERIA)

- Recent ingestion of amphetamine
- After amphetamine intake, substantial change in behavior occurs (e.g., anxiety, euphoria, hypervigilance)
- After amphetamine ingestion, two or more of the following occur:
  - Tachycardia or bradycardia
  - Pupillary dilation
  - Elevated or lowered blood pressure
  - Perspiration or chills
  - Nausea or vomiting
  - Weight loss
  - Psychomotor agitation or retardation
  - Muscular weakness, respiratory depression, chest pain, or cardiac arrhythmias
  - Confusion, seizures, dyskinesias, dystonias, or coma

AMPHETAMINE WITHDRAWAL (ACCORDING TO DSM-IV-TR CRITERIA)

- Recent decrease in amphetamine consumption that was previously quite heavy
- After cessation of amphetamine use, dysphoric mood and two or more of the following occur:
  - Fatigue
  - Unpleasant dreams
  - Sleep disturbances (insomnia or hypersomnia)
  - Increased appetite
  - Psychomotor agitation or retardation
- Symptoms cause significant social or occupational impairment

■ MISCELLANEOUS

- Structurally related to catecholamine neurotransmitters (epinephrine, norepinephrine, dopamine)
- Chronic use may produce paranoid psychosis

Amphetamine Intoxication

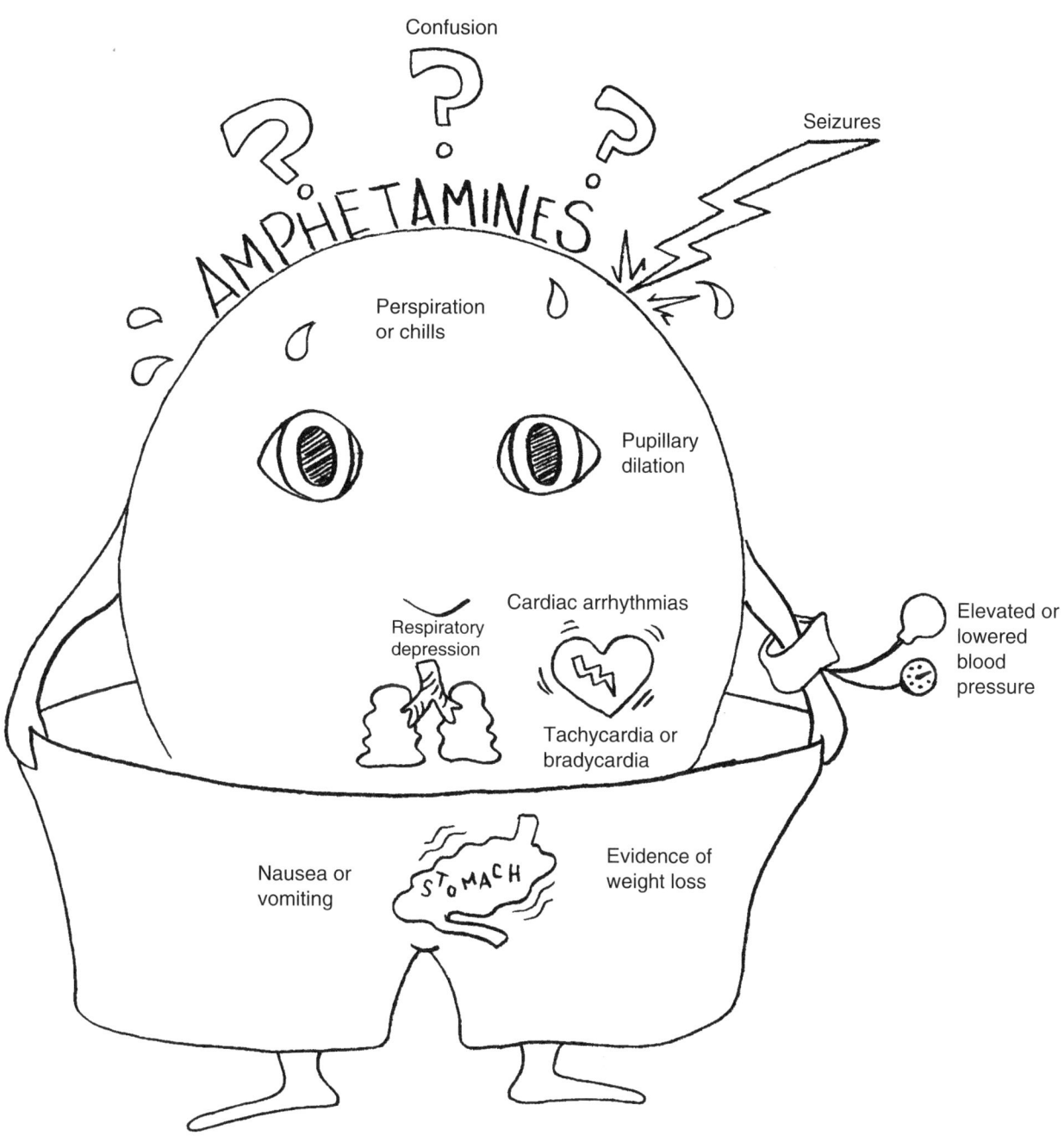

7. Substance Abuse

NOTES

CANNABIS INTOXICATION (ACCORDING TO DSM-IV-TR CRITERIA)

- Recent cannabis ingestion
- After cannabis intake, substantial change in behavior occurs (e.g., impaired motor coordination, euphoria, anxiety, sensation of slowed time, inappropriate laughter)
- Within 2 hours of cannabis use, two or more of the following occur:
  - Conjunctival injection
  - Increased appetite
  - Dry mouth
  - Tachycardia

■ MISCELLANEOUS

- Also known as marijuana or hemp
- Administered by smoking or ingestion of dried plant remnants
- Has been used medically as an antiemetic and agent to decrease intraocular pressure
- Cessation does not produce significant withdrawal symptoms

Cannabis Intoxication

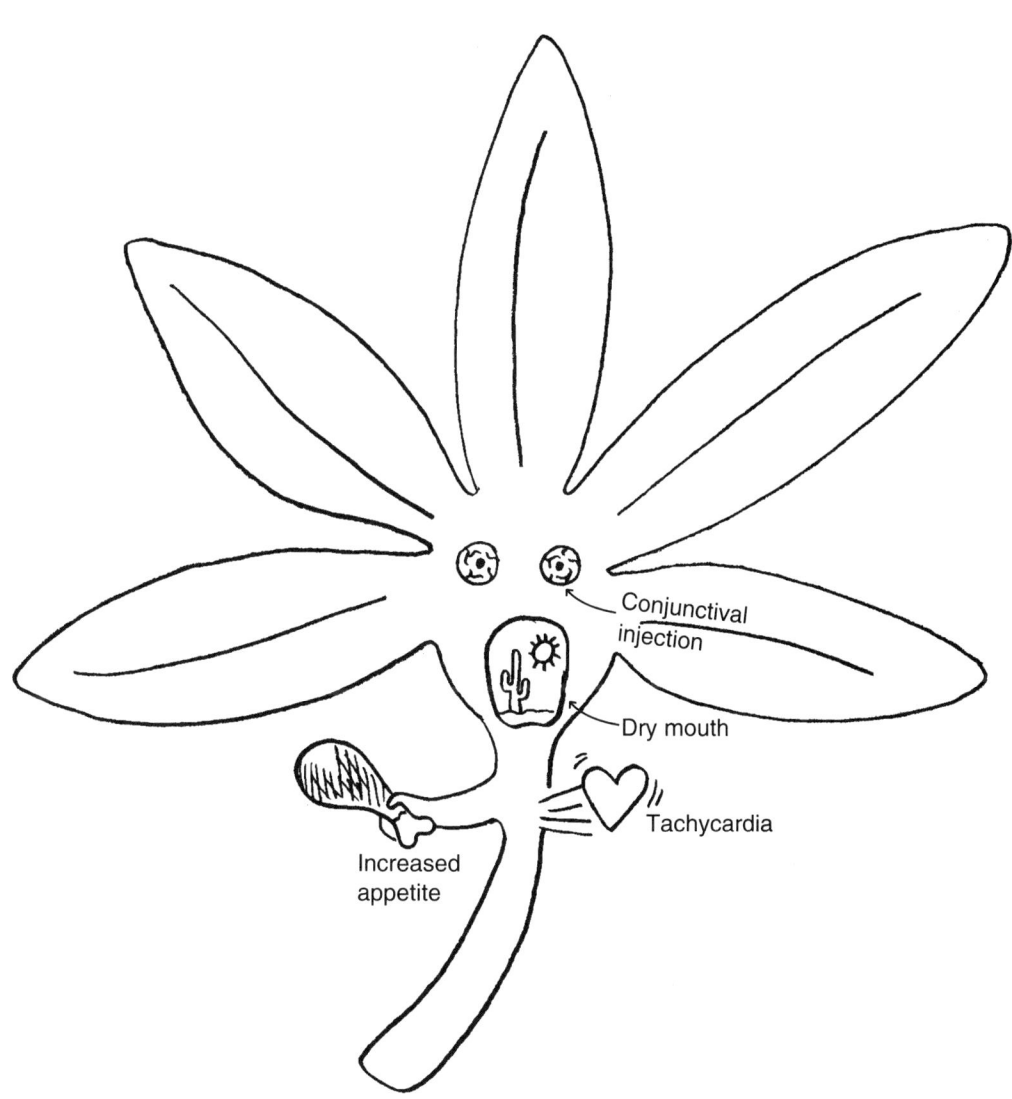

7. Substance Abuse

NOTES

COCAINE INTOXICATION (ACCORDING TO DSM-IV-TR CRITERIA)

- Recent cocaine use
- After cocaine intake, substantial change in behavior occurs (e.g., anxiety or anger; hypervigilance)
- After cocaine use, two or more of the following occur:
  - Tachycardia or bradycardia
  - Pupillary dilation
  - Elevated or lowered blood pressure
  - Perspiration or chills
  - Nausea or vomiting
  - Weight loss
  - Muscular weakness, respiratory depression, chest pain, or cardiac arrhythmias
  - Confusion, seizures, dyskinesias, dystonias, or coma

COCAINE WITHDRAWAL (ACCORDING TO DSM-IV-TR CRITERIA)

- Recent decrease in cocaine consumption that was previously quite heavy
- After cessation of cocaine use, dysphoric mood and two or more of the following occur:
  - Fatigue
  - Unpleasant dreams
  - Sleep disturbances (insomnia or hypersomnia)
  - Increased appetite
  - Psychomotor agitation or retardation
- Symptoms cause significant social or occupational impairment

■ MISCELLANEOUS

- Can be administered by being inhaled intranasally or intravenous injection of cocaine "freebase," also known as crack
- Cocaine is a local anesthetic that inhibits nerve impulses by affecting the sodium conductance of nerve cell membranes; also sympathomimetic that potentiates actions of catecholamines
- Short half-life of 1 to 2 hours
- Cocaine does not have a physiologic withdrawal syndrome, and treatment may consist of psychotherapy or behavior modification

Cocaine Intoxication

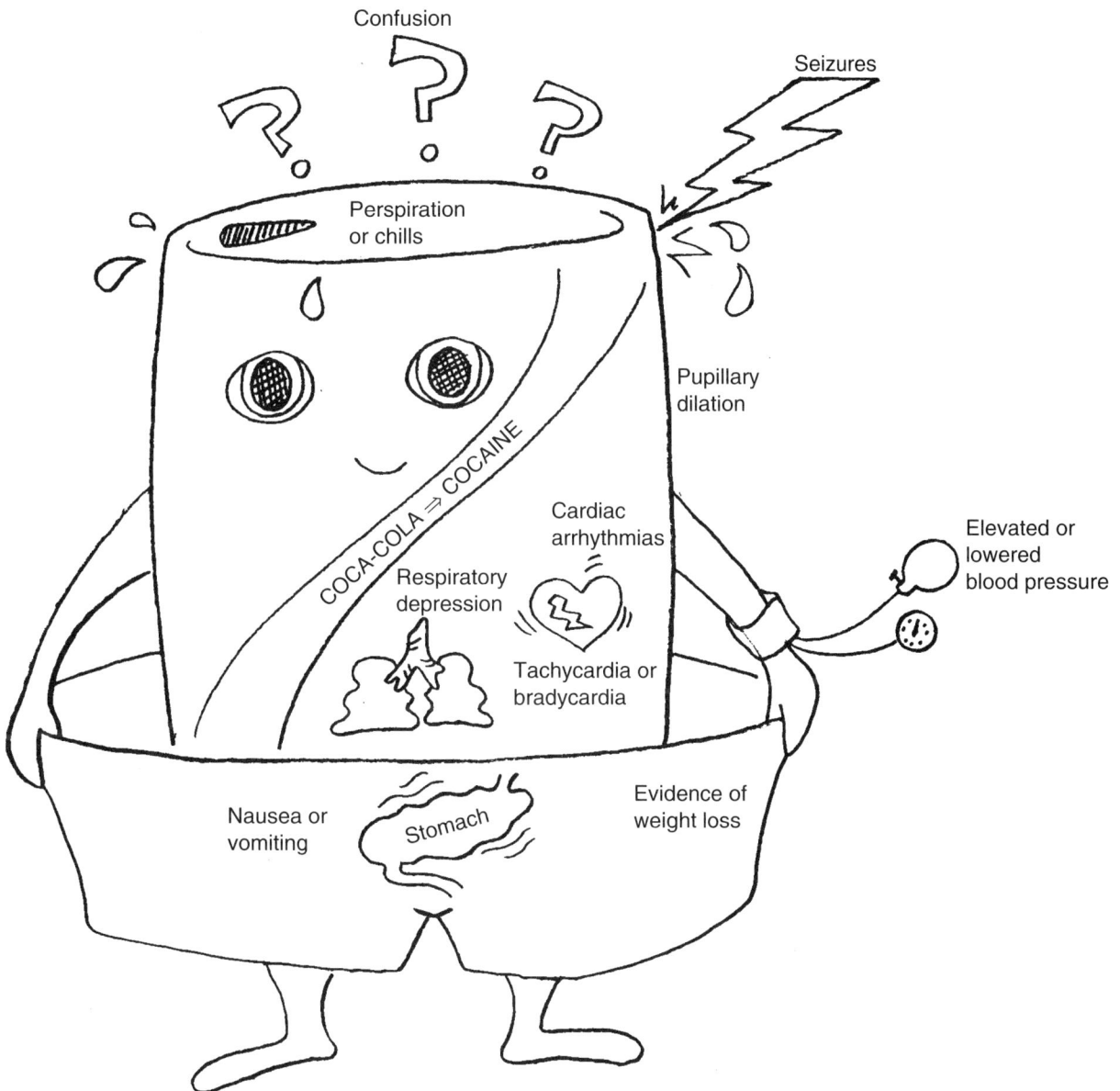

7. Substance Abuse

HALLUCINOGEN INTOXICATION (ACCORDING TO DSM-IV-TR CRITERIA)

- Recent use of hallucinogen
- After hallucinogen intake, substantial change in behavior occurs (e.g., anxiety or depression; ideas of reference; fear of losing one's mind; paranoid ideation)
- While awake and alert, perceptual disturbances occur during or after hallucinogen use (e.g., depersonalization, hallucinations)
- After hallucinogen use, two or more of the following occur:
  - Pupillary dilation
  - Tachycardia
  - Sweating
  - Palpitations
  - Blurring of vision
  - Tremors
  - Incoordination

■ MISCELLANEOUS

- Examples include lysergic acid diethylamide (LSD), mescaline, and methylenedioxyamphetamine (MDMA, ecstasy)
- Intoxication episodes are short lived (several hours), and treatment includes reducing agitation and psychosis and preventing patient from harming self or others

Hallucinogen Intoxication

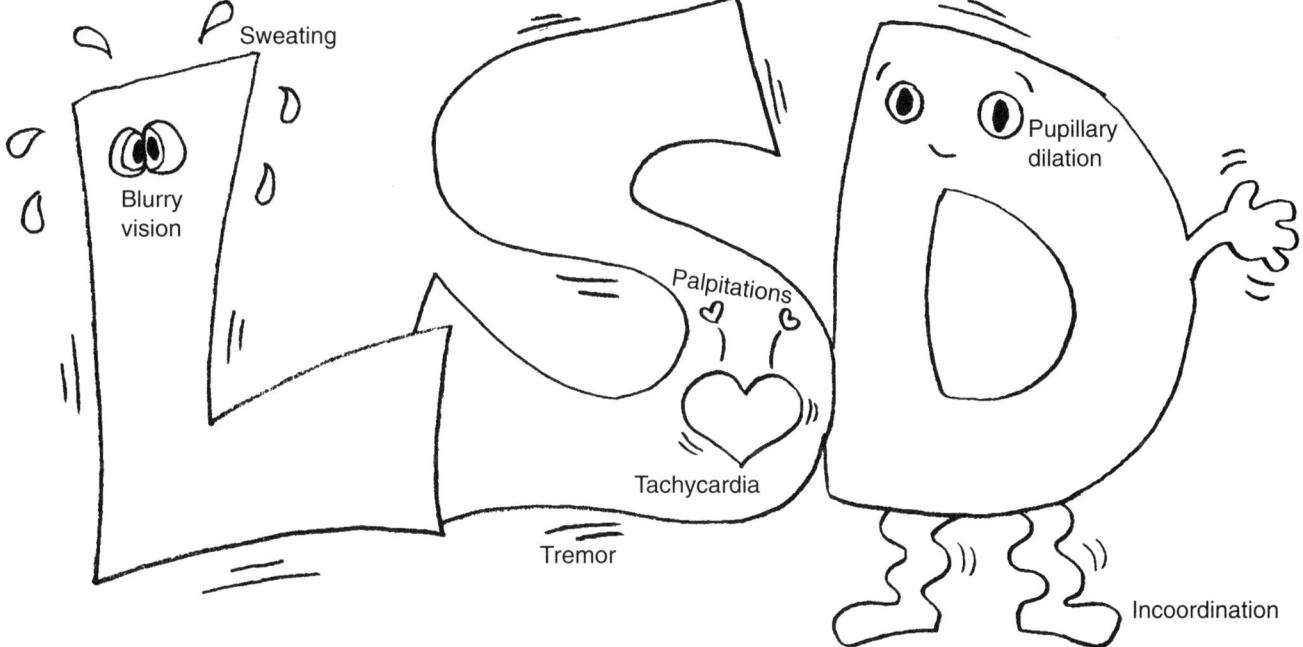

7. Substance Abuse

OPIOID INTOXICATION (ACCORDING TO DSM-IV-TR CRITERIA)

- Recent use of opioid
- After opioid intake, substantial change in behavior occurs (e.g., initial euphoria followed by apathy)
- After opioid use, pupillary constriction (however, pupillary dilation can occur following anoxia from extreme overdose) and one or more of the following occurs:
  - Drowsiness or coma
  - Slurred speech
  - Memory or attention impairment

OPIOID WITHDRAWAL (ACCORDING TO DSM-IV-TR CRITERIA)

- Recent decrease in opioid consumption that was previously quite heavy or use of opioid antagonist after period of opioid use
- Within minutes to days after opioid cessation, three or more of the following occur:
  - Dysphoric mood
  - Nausea or vomiting
  - Muscle aches
  - Lacrimation or rhinorrhea
  - Pupillary dilation, piloerection, or sweating
  - Diarrhea
  - Yawning
  - Fever
  - Insomnia
- Symptoms cause significant social or occupational impairment

■ MISCELLANEOUS

- Stimulates receptors for endogenous hormones, endorphins, enkephalins, and dynorphins
- Opioid receptors include mu, kappa, delta, and epsilon
- Examples of opioids include morphine, heroin, and methadone, which react with mu receptors, which are responsible for analgesia, euphoria, and respiratory depression
- Opioid overdose is life-threatening (coma and respiratory suppression), and emergency respiratory and cardiovascular support may be required; naloxone (an opioid antagonist) will reverse coma and respiratory suppression
- Opioid withdrawal is not life-threatening (characterized by increased sympathetic nervous system activity); clonidine may be used to suppress symptoms of withdrawal, and methadone is most commonly used for detoxification

Opioid Intoxication

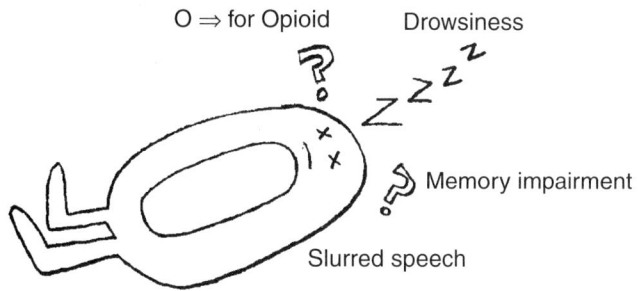

Opioid Withdrawal

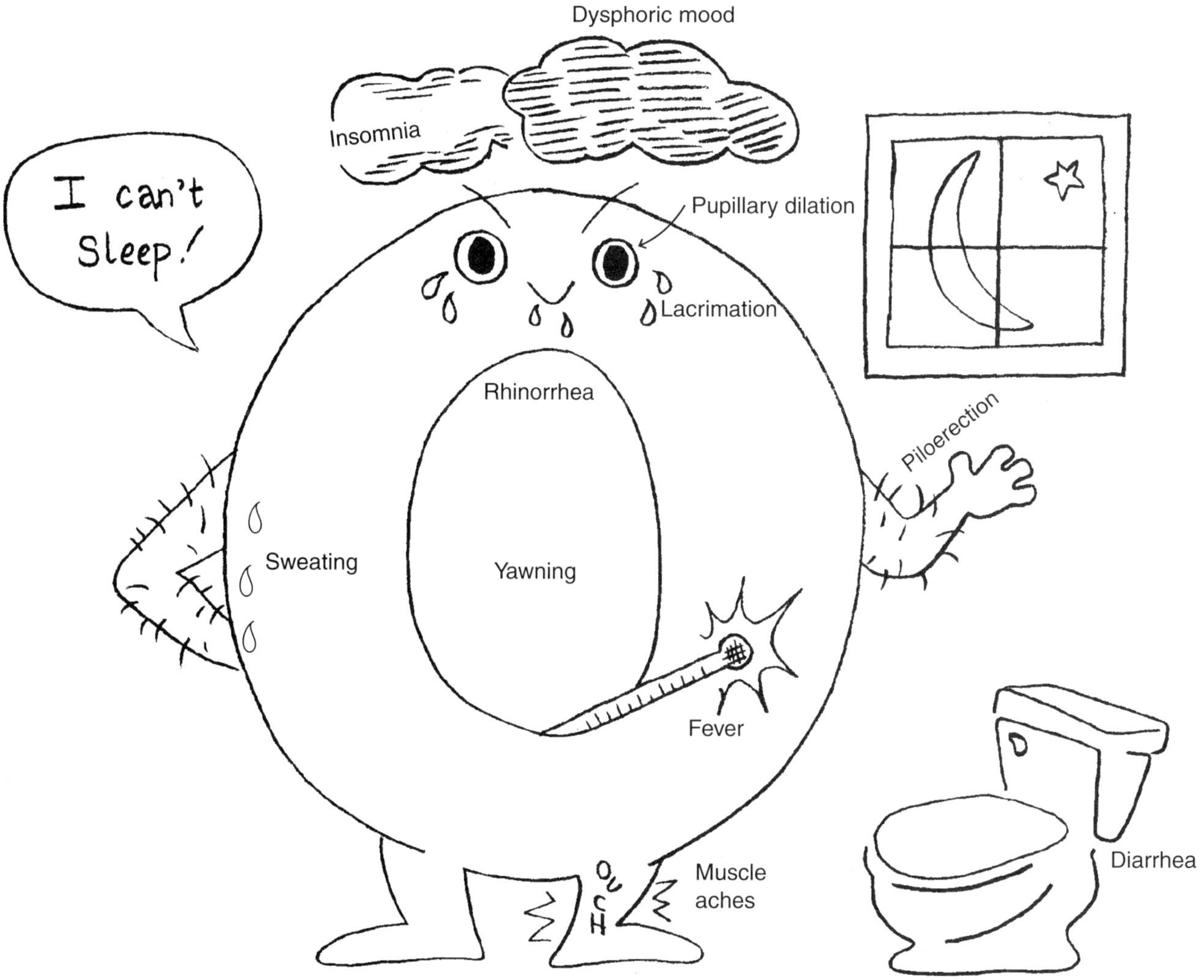

7. Substance Abuse

SEDATIVE, HYPNOTIC, OR ANXIOLYTIC INTOXICATION (ACCORDING TO DSM-IV-TR CRITERIA)

- Recent use of sedative, hypnotic, or anxiolytic
- After sedative, hypnotic, or anxiolytic intake, substantial change in behavior occurs (e.g., inappropriate sexual or aggressive behavior, mood ability)
- After alcohol ingestion, one or more of the following occurs:
  - Slurred speech
  - Incoordination
  - Unsteady gait
  - Nystagmus
  - Memory impairment
  - Stupor or coma

SEDATIVE, HYPNOTIC, OR ANXIOLYTIC WITHDRAWAL (ACCORDING TO DSM-IV-TR CRITERIA)

- Recent decrease in sedative, hypnotic, or anxiolytic consumption that was previously quite heavy
- After cessation of sedative, hypnotic, or anxiolytic intake, two or more of the following occur:
  - Autonomic hyperactivity
  - Increased hand tremor
  - Insomnia
  - Nausea/vomiting
  - Transient hallucinations
  - Psychomotor agitation
  - Anxiety
  - Grand mal seizures
- Symptoms cause significant social or occupational impairment

■ MISCELLANEOUS

- Examples include barbiturates, benzodiazepines, and nonbarbiturate sedative hypnotics (methaqualone)
- Gamma-hydroxybutyrate (GHB) is illegal in the United States and has been used in "date rape" scenarios
- These drugs interact with the gamma-aminobutyric acid (GABA)-chloride channel receptor (i.e., benzodiazepines facilitate GABA binding to its receptor, therefore enhancing the inhibitory effects of GABA)
- Treatment of intoxication includes support of vital functions; flumazenil (benzodiazepine antagonist) can be used for benzodiazepine overdose but has minimal effects when used with other sedatives, hypnotics, or anxiolytics

Sedative, Hypnotic, or Anxiolytic Intoxication

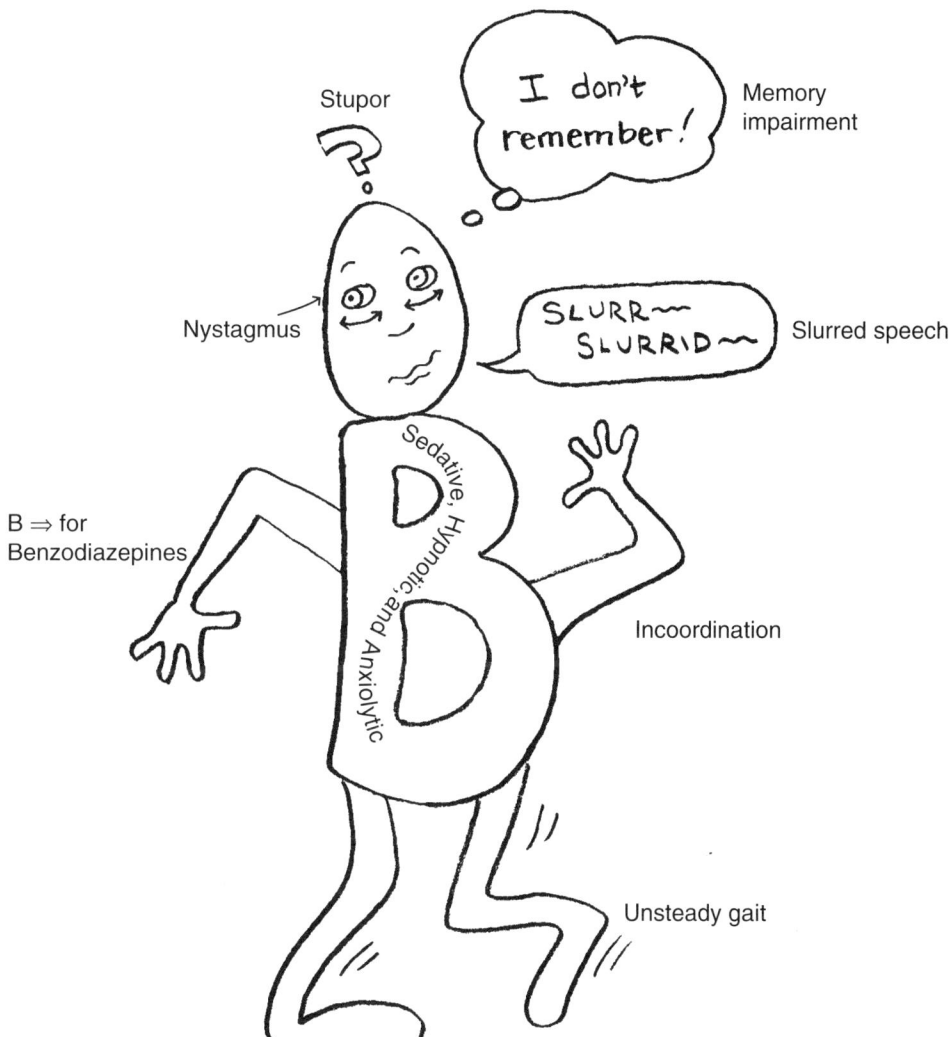

8. Eating Disorders

NOTES

EATING DISORDERS: ANOREXIA NERVOSA

- DSM IV criteria include:
  - Patient's body weight is not maintained above 85% of expected weight for age and height
    - ⇒ scale
  - Fear of gaining weight or being overweight even though patient remains underweight
  - Denial of seriousness of patient's low weight
  - Preoccupation with body size and weight
  - Amenorrhea is present for three cycles in postmenarchal females
    - ⇒ tampons in trash
- Classification of anorexia nervosa:
  - Restricting Type involves excessive dieting and exercise; binging and purging are not present
    - excessive exercise
    - ⇒ lifting dumbbell
  - Binge Eating or Purging Type may include excessive dieting and exercise; purging may involve vomiting, abuse of laxatives, diuretics, or enemas
    - purging ⇒ vomit
- Prevalence in females is 0.5% to 1.0%
- More than 90% of patients with anorexia nervosa are female
- Average age of onset is 17 years; onset is rare after age 40
- Delay of menarche may occur in premenarchal females
- Increased incidence in first-degree relatives and a higher concordance in monozygotic twins
- Anorexia nervosa often involves obsessive-compulsive symptoms, including calorie counting and food hoarding
  - calorie counting ⇒ counting with fingers
- Often coexists with major depressive disorder
  - ⇒ sad and crying
- The long-term mortality rate is 10% secondary to suicide or medical complications
  - ⇒ tombstone
- Differential diagnosis includes major depression, medical conditions (e.g., malignancies, AIDS), social phobia of eating in public, body dysmorphic disorder, and bulimia nervosa
- Anorexia nervosa is differentiated from bulimia nervosa by the presence of low weight in anorexia and the ability to maintain weight in bulimia
- Treatment includes:
  - Psychotherapy, behavioral therapy, family therapy, and group therapy
  - Treatment programs may include monitoring of oral intake, body weight, and electrolytes
  - Pharmacotherapy often includes selective serotonin reuptake inhibitors (SSRIs) for coexisting depression

Anorexia Nervosa

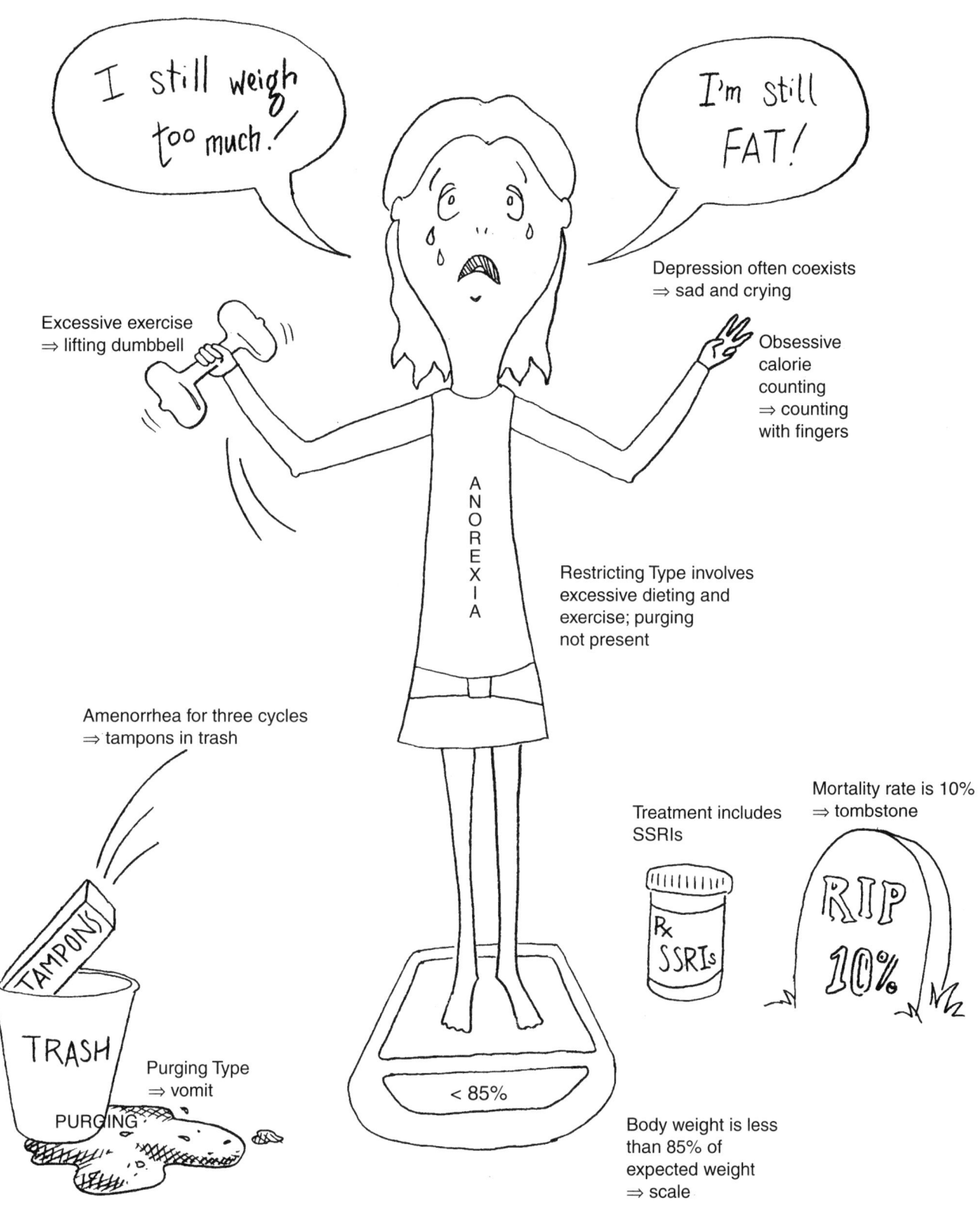

8. Eating Disorders

EATING DISORDERS: BULIMIA NERVOSA

⇒ bull eating

- DSM IV criteria include:
  - Patient engages in recurrent episodes of binging, defined as eating an increased amount of food within 2 hours
    - binging ⇒ chips and candy
  - Patient engages in behavior to prevent weight gain (e.g., exercise abuse, vomiting, ipecac-induced vomiting, laxative abuse, diuretics, and enemas)
    - exercise abuse ⇒ lifting dumbbell
  - Patient has a feeling of lack of self-control over eating during binging episode
  - The above occur twice a week on average for three months
- Classification of bulimia nervosa:
  - Purging Type: Patient regularly uses self-induced vomiting, laxatives, and enemas
    - purging ⇒ vomit
  - Nonpurging Type: Patient regularly exercises and restricts intake but does not vomit or use laxatives or enemas
- Bulimic patients maintain their expected body weight for age
  - ⇒ scale
- Patient's self-evaluation is overly influenced by body shape and weight
- Prevalence is 1% to 3% in females of adolescent and young adult age and 0.1% to 0.3% in males
- In bulimic patients, there is an increased incidence of borderline personality disorder and substance abuse
- Purging is often associated with poor dentition caused by acidity of vomit Purging is also associated with dehydration, electrolyte abnormalities, and esophageal rupture
- Bulimic patients tend to hide their behavior from families and doctors because of embarrassment
- Death rarely occurs in bulimia
  - ⇒ crossed-out tombstone
- Treatment includes:
  - Cognitive behavioral therapy used to improve body image
  - Psychotherapy to influence eating behavior
  - Pharmacotherapy includes selective serotonin reuptake inhibitors (SSRIs) like fluoxetine (Prozac) to reduce binging and purging

■ MEDICAL COMPLICATIONS OF EATING DISORDERS

- Vomiting
  - Poor dentition caused by acidity of vomit
  - Parotid gland enlargement
  - Esophageal rupture
  - Metabolic alkalosis
  - Hypokalemia
  - Hypochloremia
  - Cardiac arrhythmias caused by electrolyte abnormalities
  - Aspiration pneumonia
- Laxative abuse
  - Dehydration
  - Metabolic acidosis
- Diuretic abuse
  - Dehydration
  - Metabolic alkalosis
  - Cardiac arrhythmias caused by electrolyte abnormalities
- Ipecac toxicity
  - Cardiomyopathy
- Starvation
  - Cold intolerance
  - Anemia
  - Leukopenia
  - Osteoporosis
  - Lanugo hair
  - Dry skin

Bulimia Nervosa

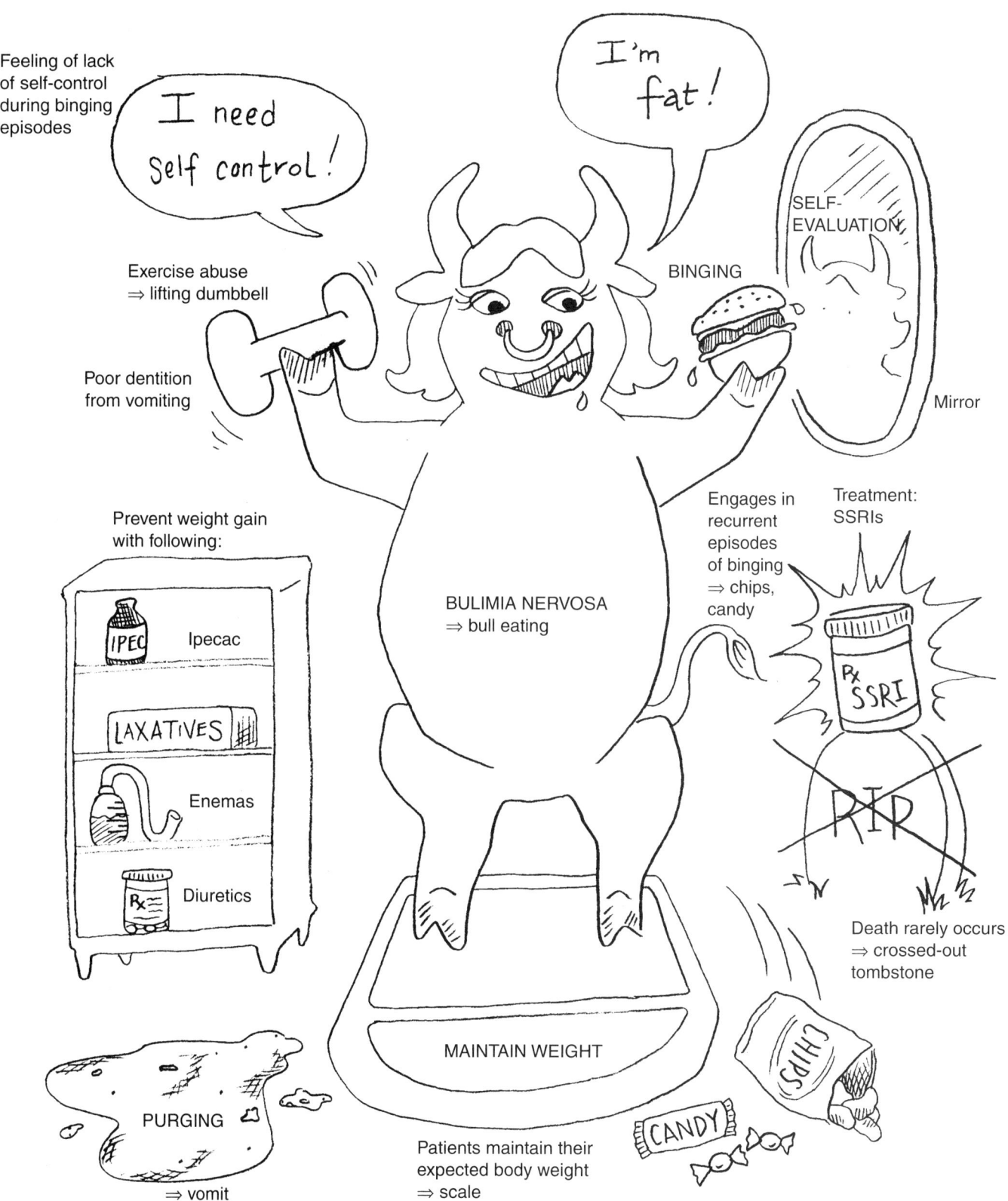

9. Dissociative Disorders

DISSOCIATIVE DISORDERS: DISSOCIATIVE AMNESIA

- Characterized by an inability to remember personal information
    - ⇒ Where was I born?
    - ⇒ Do I have children?
    - ⇒ What is my career?
- More common with trauma exposure (e.g., war, assault, natural disaster, or accident)
- Not caused by a medical or mental condition (e.g., head trauma, dementia)
- Different types include:
    - Generalized Amnesia: Memory loss continues throughout life
    - Localized Amnesia: Memory loss for a specific time interval
        - ⇒ time interval = clock
    - Continuous Amnesia: Memory loss from a specific point in time
    - Selective Amnesia: Inability to remember only some information

Dissociative Amnesia

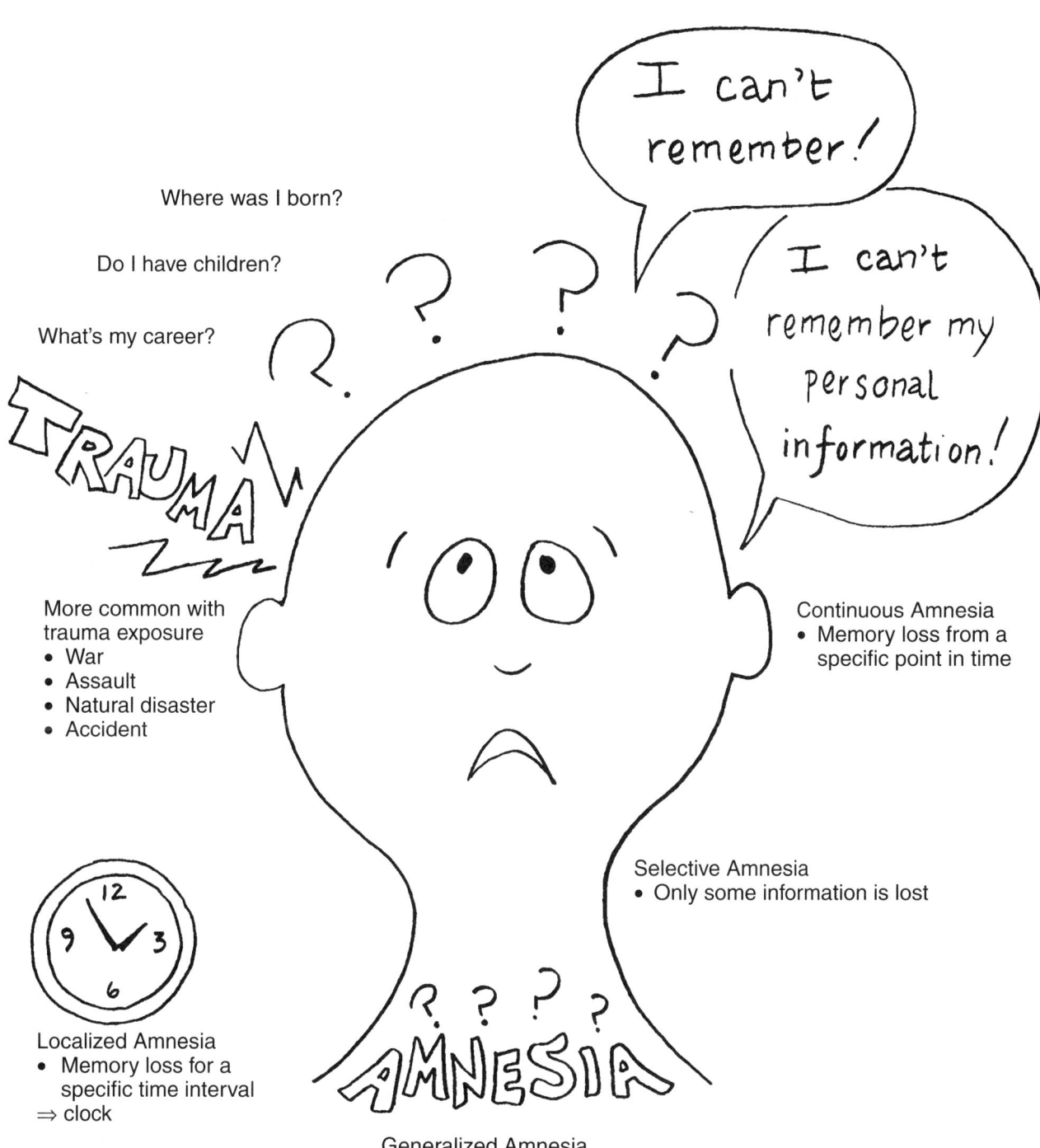

9. Dissociative Disorders

DISSOCIATIVE DISORDERS: DISSOCIATIVE FUGUE

- Characterized by identity amnesia
  ⇒ "Who am I?"
- Includes sudden travel away from home
  ⇒ car driving away from home
- History of alcohol use and stress common
  ⇒ beer, wine, and stress at home
- Can assume a new identity in the new location
- Patients usually do not realize they have assumed a new identity

Dissociative Fugue

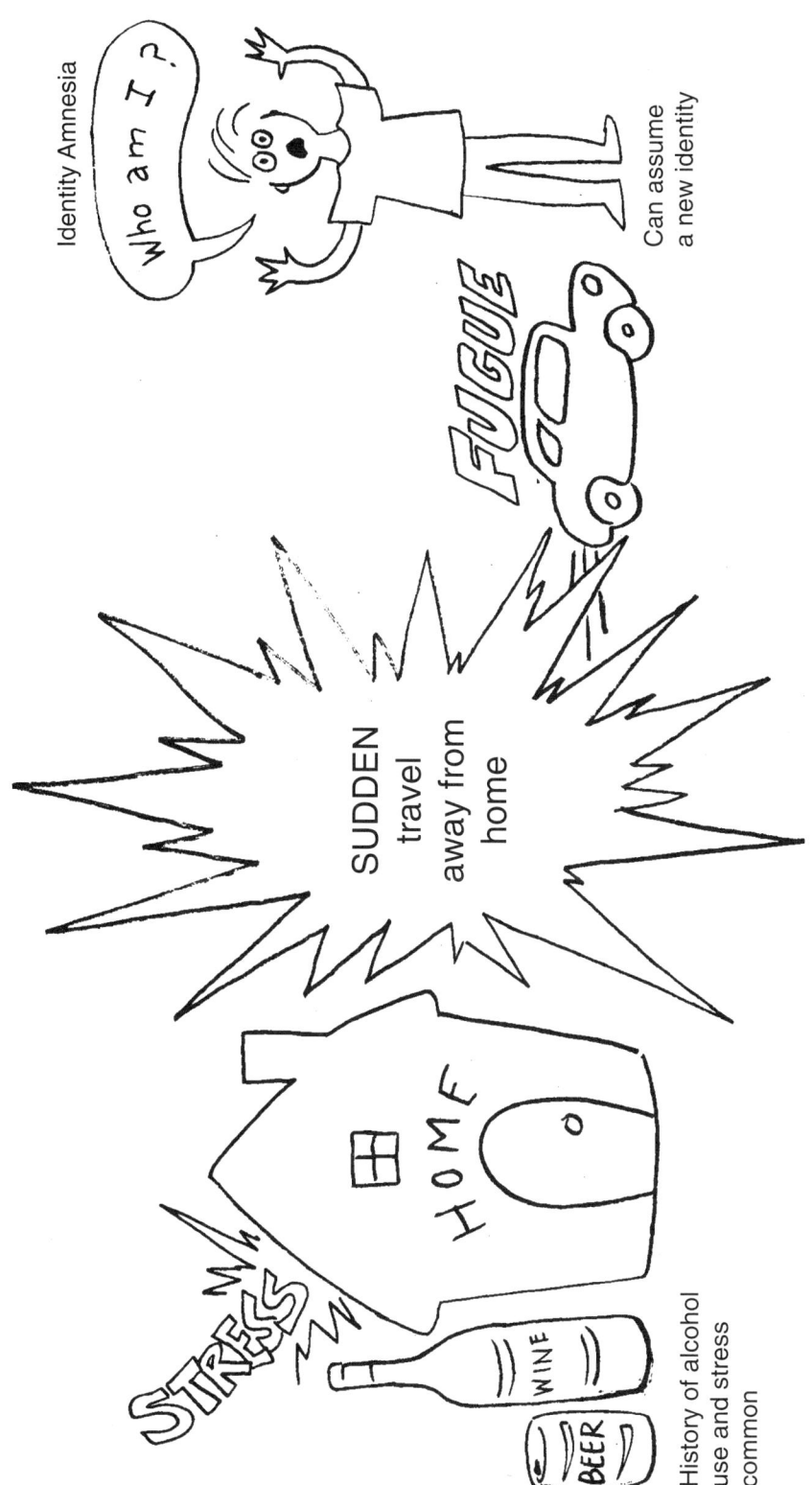

9. Dissociative Disorders

DISSOCIATIVE DISORDERS: DISSOCIATIVE IDENTITY DISORDER

- Also known as multiple personality disorder
- Characterized by the presence of at least two separate personalities
    - ⇒ two separate personalities (a teacher and a dancer) holding up two fingers
- One personality usually dominates over the other personalities
- Often have amnesia
    - ⇒ "I don't remember"
- More common in women
- The separate personalities may be of different ages and genders
- History of abuse common
    - ⇒ abuse = hanger hitting leg

Dissociative Identity Disorder

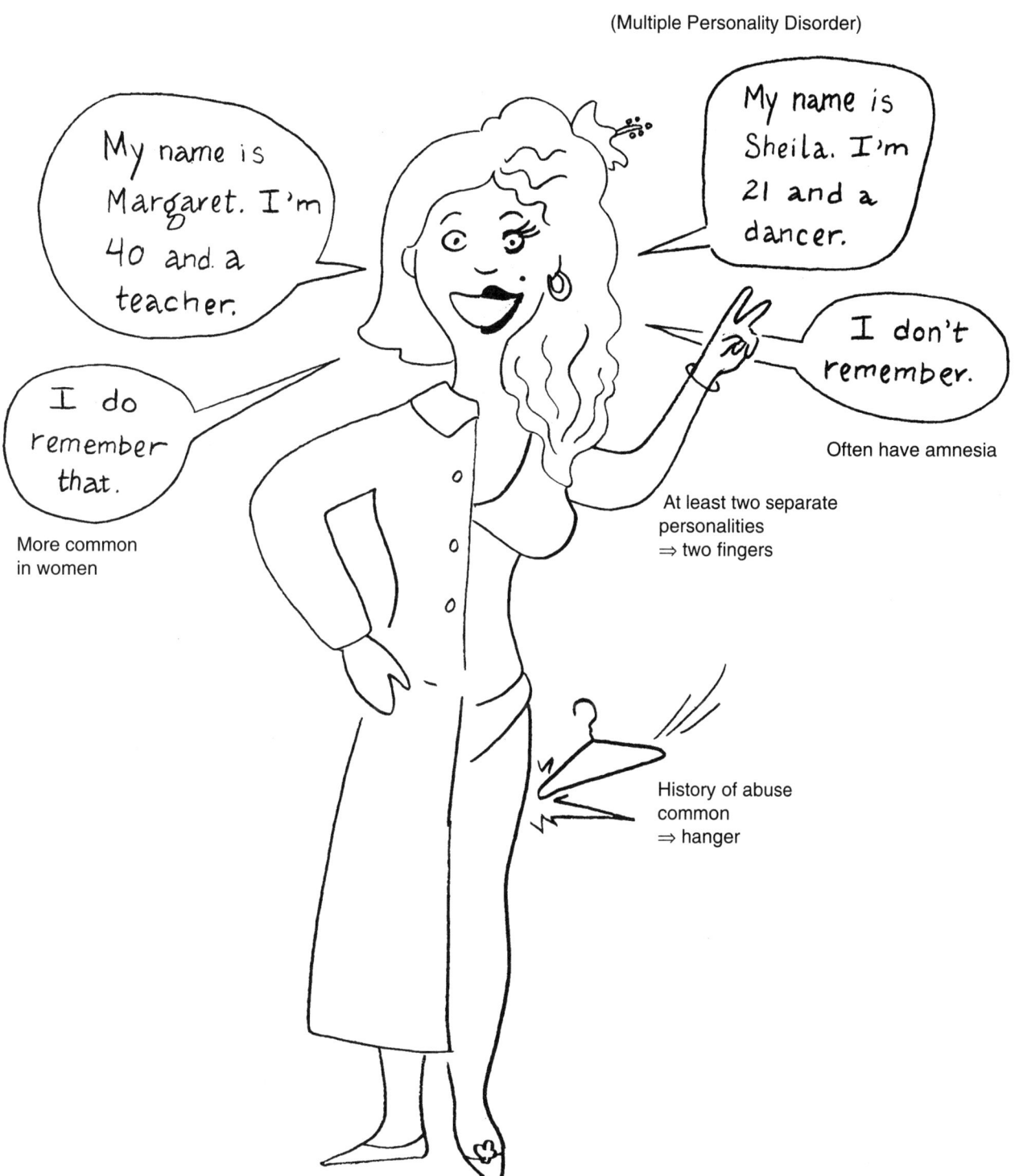

9. Dissociative Disorders

NOTES

DISSOCIATIVE DISORDERS: DEPERSONALIZATION DISORDER

- Characterized by a constant or recurrent feeling of detachment
    - ⇒ person floating over bed watching oneself
    - ⇒ "I feel outside of myself!"
- Patients are aware the feeling of detachment is not reality
    - ⇒ "I know this is NOT reality."
- Onset occurs at 15 to 30 years of age
- Associated with severe stress
    - ⇒ Stress hitting bed
- Treatment includes anxiolytics and selective serotonin reuptake inhibitors (SSRIs)

Depersonalization Disorder

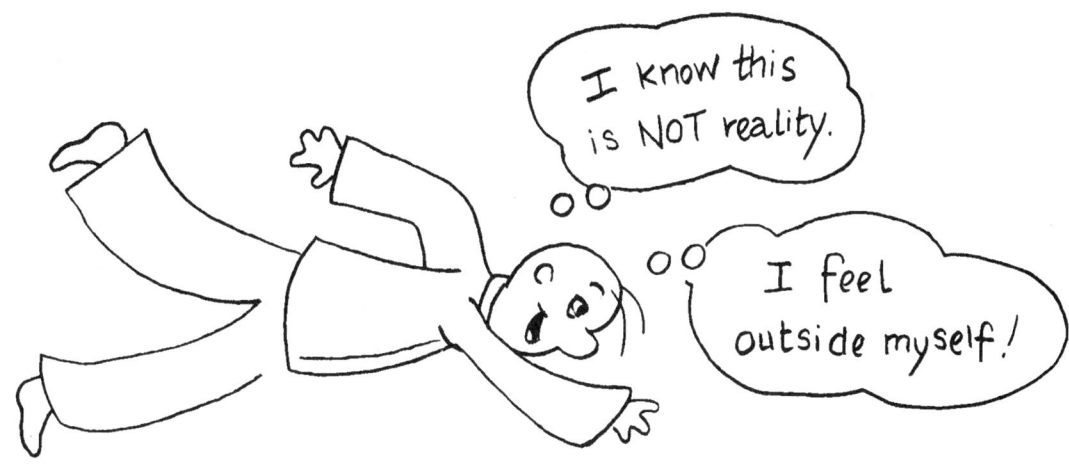
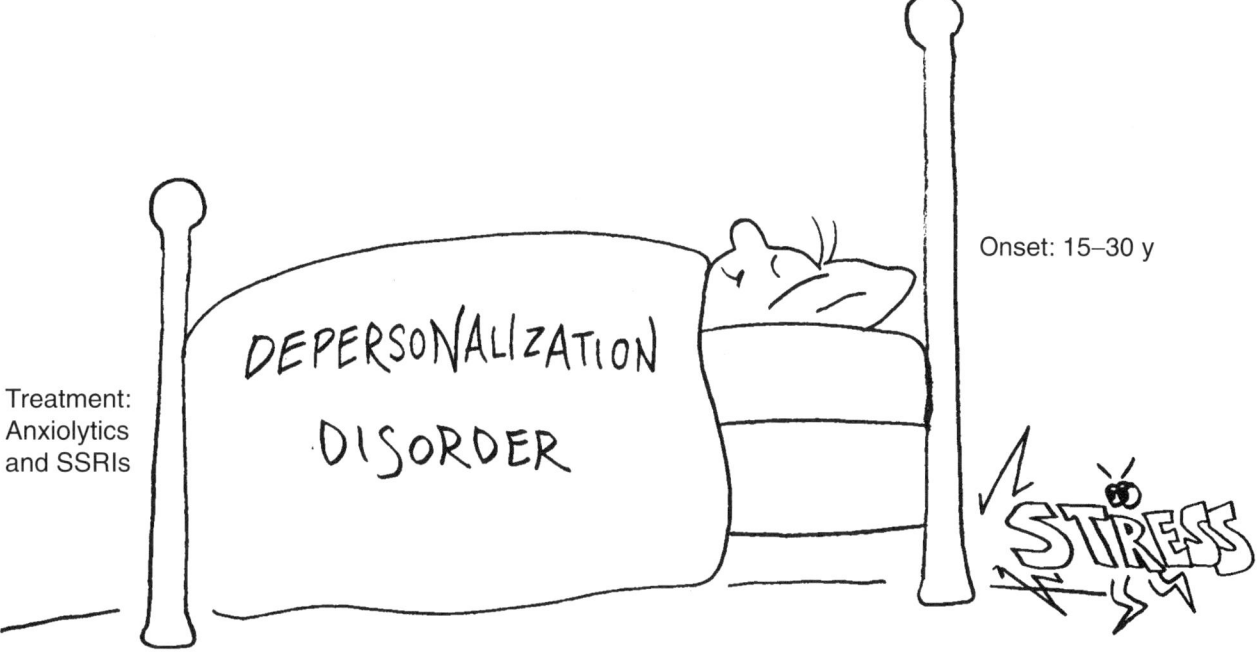

10. Psychosexual Disorders

SEXUAL RESPONSE CYCLE

- Desire Stage:
  - Involves the initial urge to have sex
- Excitement Stage:
  - The initial physiologic response to arousal
  - In men, the penis becomes erect.
  - In women, the labia and clitoris swell and the vagina lubricates.
- Plateau Stage:
  - In men, the testes enlarge and move upward.
  - In women, the outer vagina contracts while the inner section enlarges.
- Orgasm Stage:
  - In men, seminal fluid is ejaculated.
  - In women, the uterus and vagina contract.
- In all of the above stages, pulse, respiration rate, and blood pressure all increase.
  - ⇒ heart shooting upward
- Resolution Stage:
  - Involves muscle relaxation and a return to a normal physiologic state
    ⇒ heart falling down
  - In men, includes a refractory period when restimulation will not occur. Women have a short to no refractory period.

Sexual Response Cycle

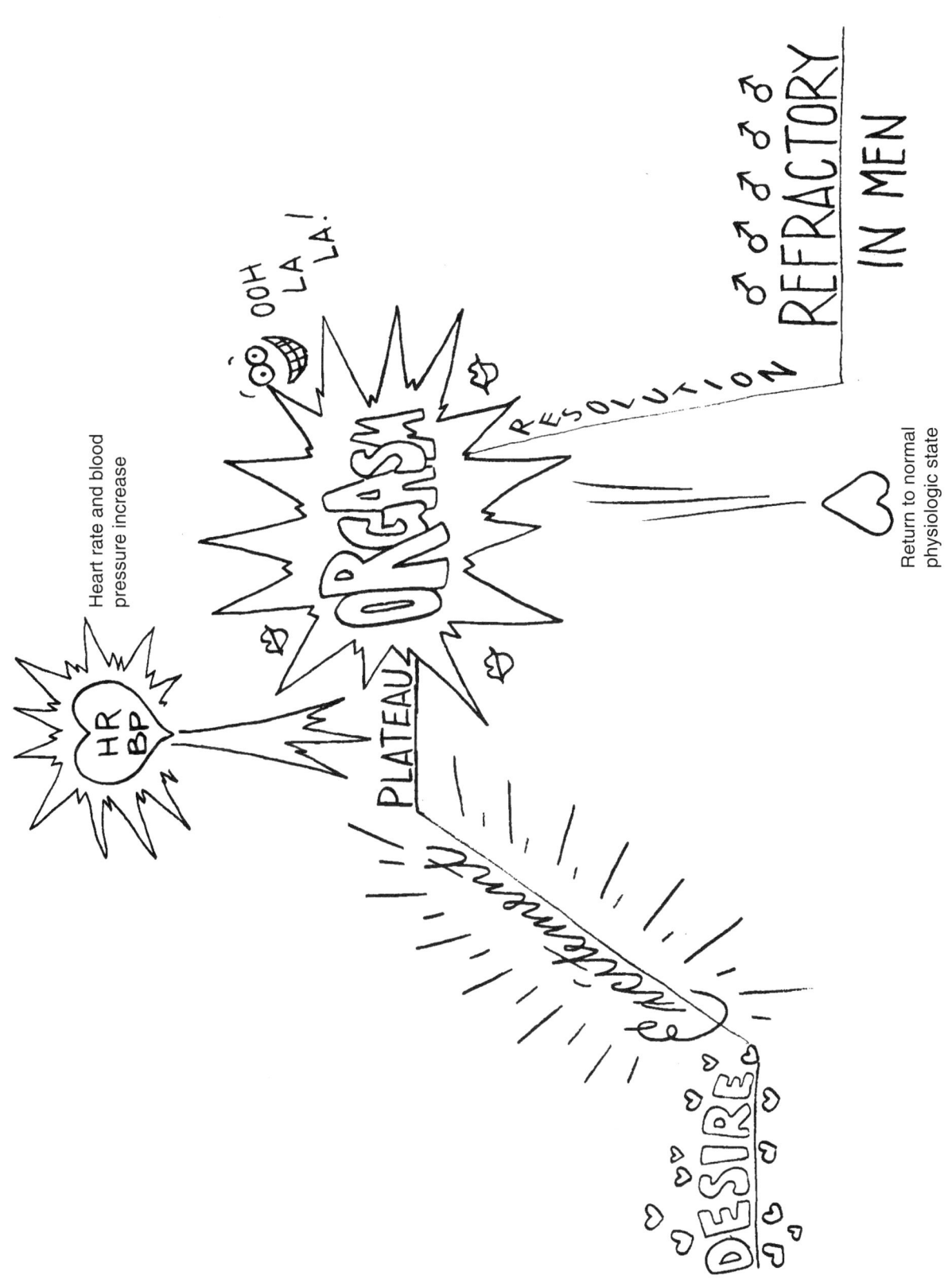

10. Psychosexual Disorders

SEXUAL DYSFUNCTIONS

- Sexual desire disorders:
  - **Hypoactive sexual desire disorder**
    - Decreased or absent desire or interest in sexual activity
      ⇒ "I have no desire!"
  - **Sexual aversion disorder**
    - Aversion to sexual activity with another person
      ⇒ "Don't kiss me! Don't touch my genitals!"
- Sexual arousal disorders (excitement phase disorder):
  - **Female sexual arousal disorder**
    - Unable to produce vaginal lubrication and become aroused with physical stimulation, although interested in sexual activity
  - **Male erectile disorder** (impotence)
    - Inability to obtain or maintain an erection
      ⇒ "My penis is not working!"
- Orgasmic disorders (orgasm phase disorder, normal excitement phase):
  - **Female or male orgasmic disorder**
    - Inability to reach orgasm despite adequate arousal and stimulation
      ⇒ "I'm aroused, but I can't reach orgasm!"
  - **Premature ejaculation**
    - Early ejaculation occurs with little stimulation
      ⇒ "Oops! Sorry!"
- Sexual pain disorders:
  - **Dyspareunia**
    - Pelvic pain associated with intercourse
    - Not caused by a medical condition; normal pelvic exam
      ⇒ "Ouch! That hurts!"
  - **Vaginismus**
    - Painful spasm of the outer vagina with attempted penetration
      ⇒ "Ow! My vagina is in a SPASM!"

Sexual Dysfunctions

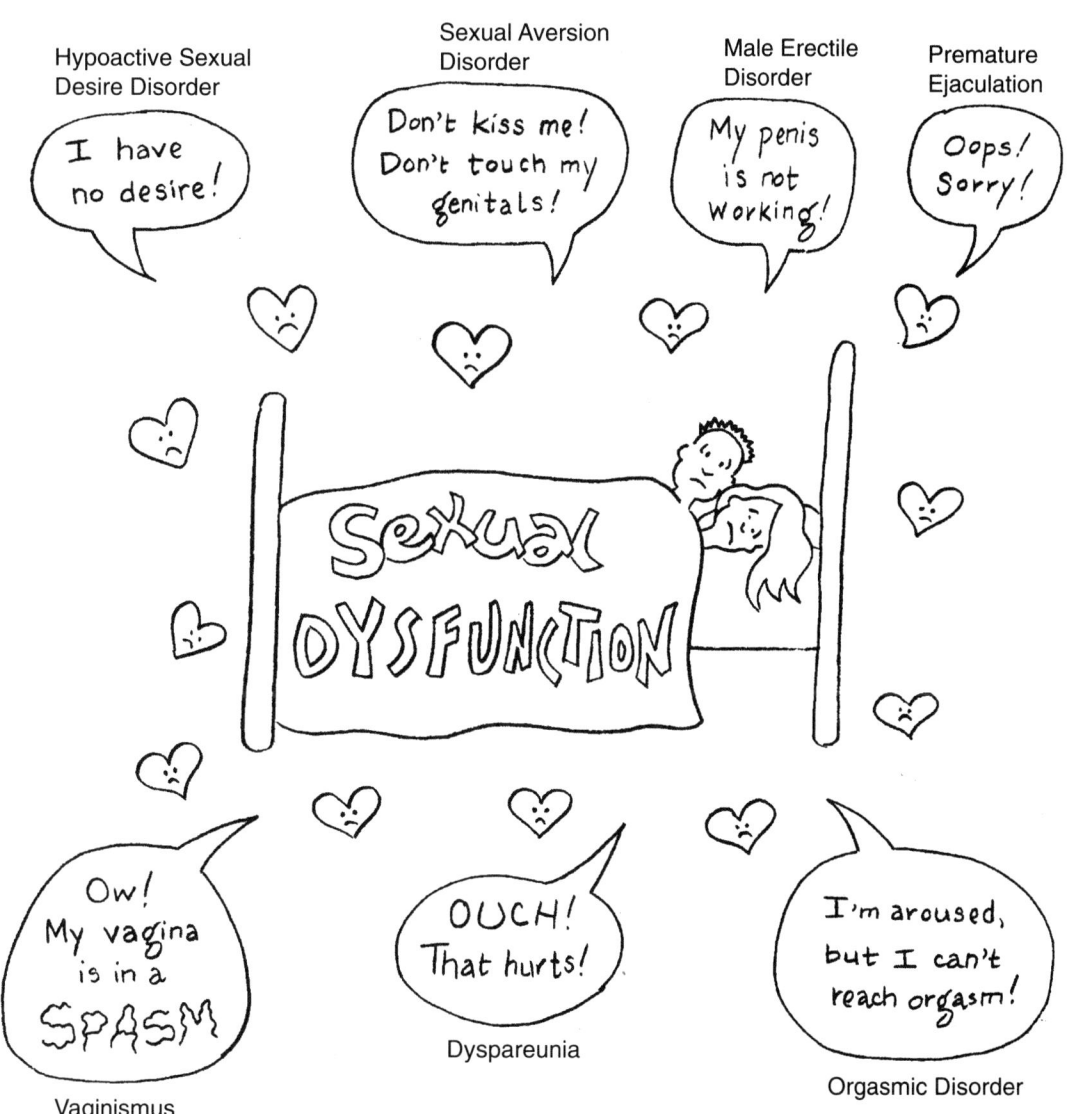

11. Paraphilias

PARAPHILIAS

- Preoccupation with using unusual objects and unusual behavior for sexual stimulation and satisfaction
- Occurs over six months and impairs social and occupational functioning
- Almost exclusive to men
- **Exhibitionism:** Revealing of one's genitals to strangers in order to shock them
- **Fetishism:** The use of inanimate (nonliving) objects for sexual pleasure
- **Transvestic Fetishism:** Exclusive to heterosexual men; involves cross-dressing for sexual arousal
- **Frotteurism:** Touching or rubbing (usually genitals) against an unsuspecting individual for sexual pleasure
- **Pedophilia:** An individual has fantasies or acts on sexual urges involving children younger than 13; individual is at least 16 years old and 5 years older than the child
- **Sexual Masochism:** Individual is sexually aroused by being humiliated, beaten, or made to suffer
- **Sexual Sadism:** Individual is sexually aroused by inflicting pain and humiliation on sexual partner
- **Voyeurism:** Individual is sexually aroused by observing in unsuspecting individual disrobing or involved in sexual activity
- **Treatment:** Pharmacologic (antiandrogens and female sex hormones) and psychotherapy

Paraphilias

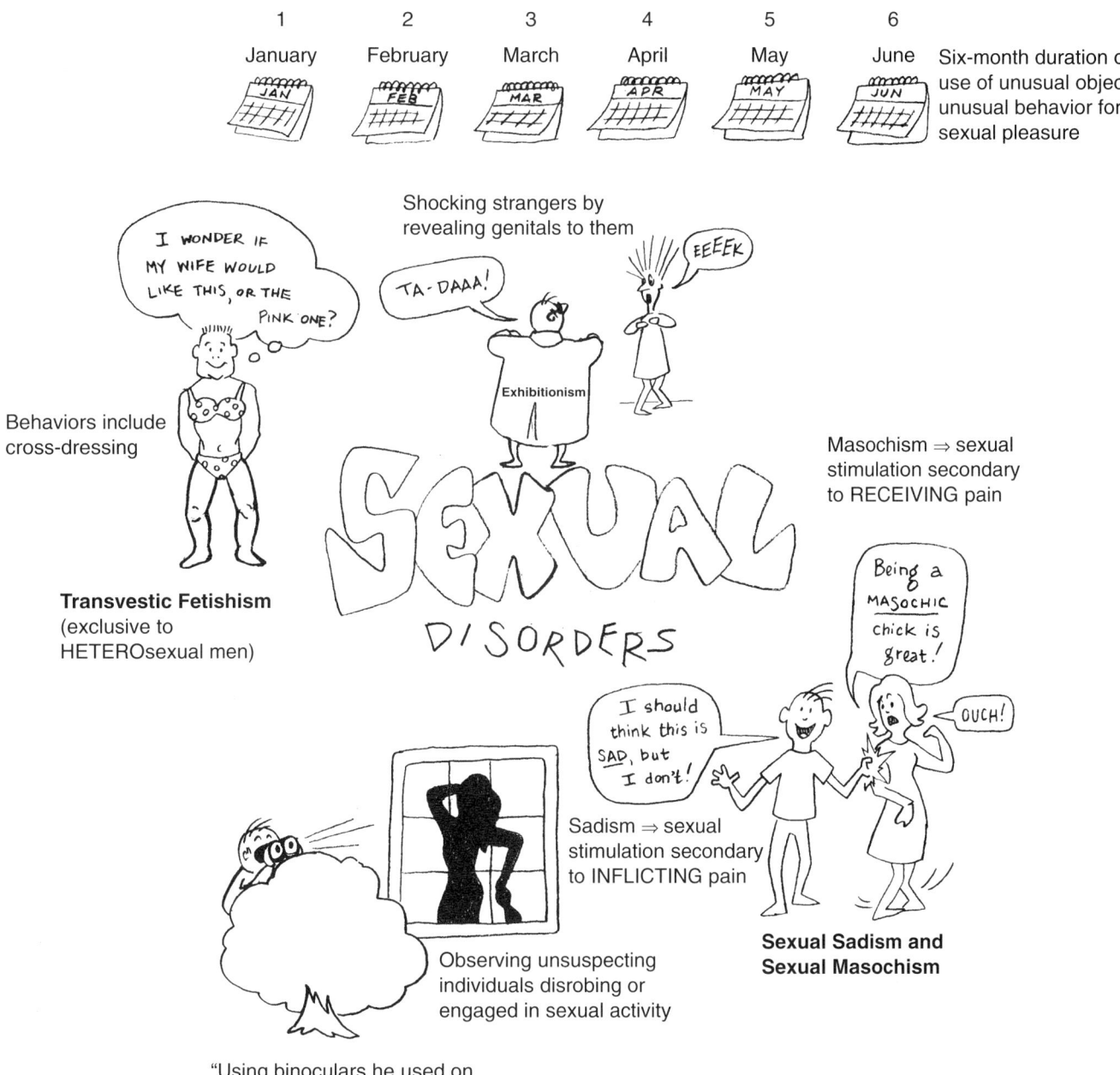

12. Phobias

NOTES

AGORAPHOBIA
- Not codable disorder according to DSM-IV
- Agoraphobia is considered to occur with other disorders such as panic disorder.
- Individuals with agoraphobia fear places or situations in which escape would be difficult or impossible (e.g., riding in trains, buses, or automobiles, standing in crowds, or being on bridges).
- Agoraphobic individuals avoid these situations to the best of their ability.

Agoraphobia

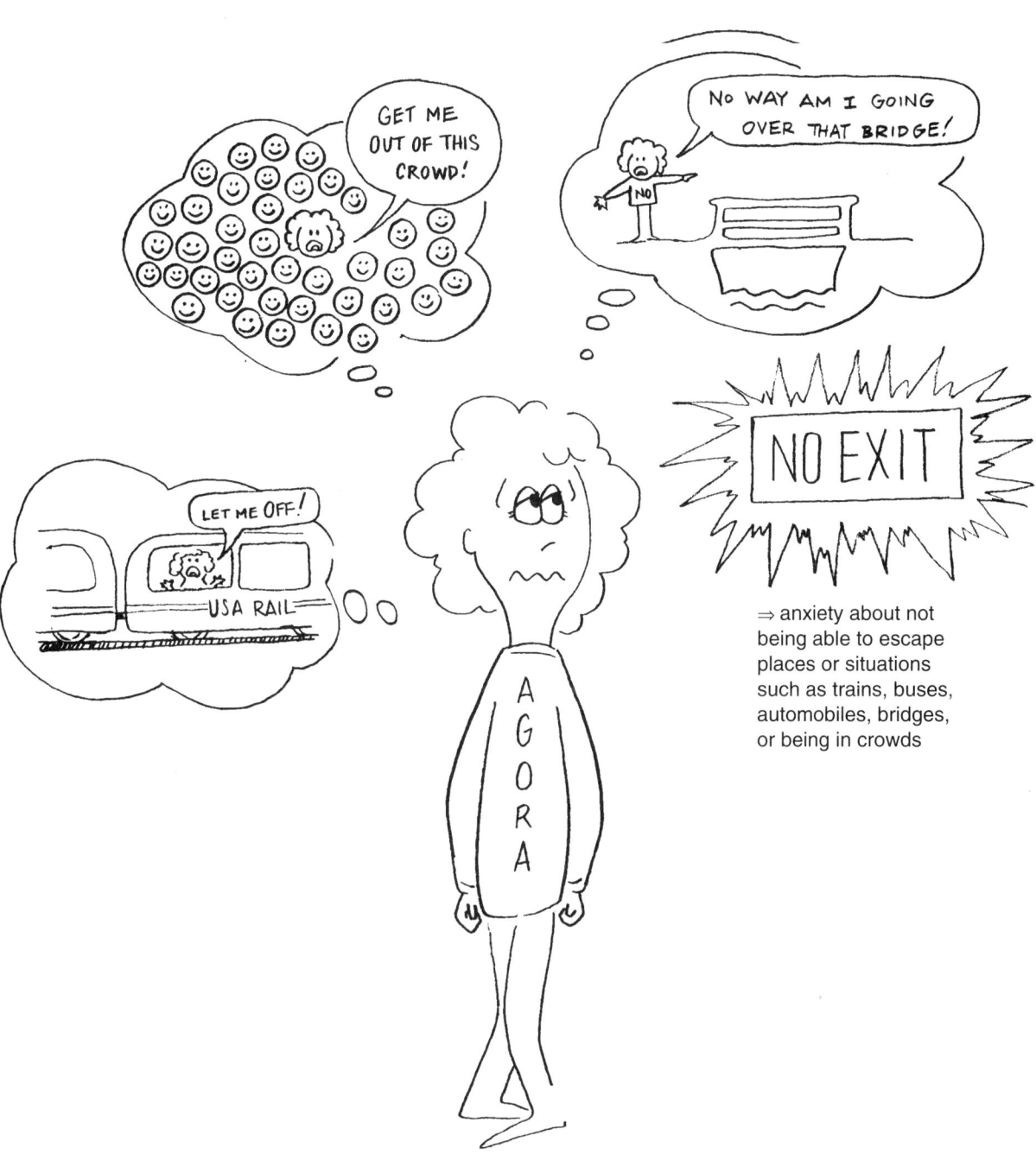

⇒ anxiety about not being able to escape places or situations such as trains, buses, automobiles, bridges, or being in crowds

12. Phobias

SOCIAL PHOBIA
- Persistent fear of social or performance situations, especially when exposed to unfamiliar individuals or places, according to DSM-IV-TR
- Individual anxious about doing something embarrassing or being criticized by others

Social Phobia

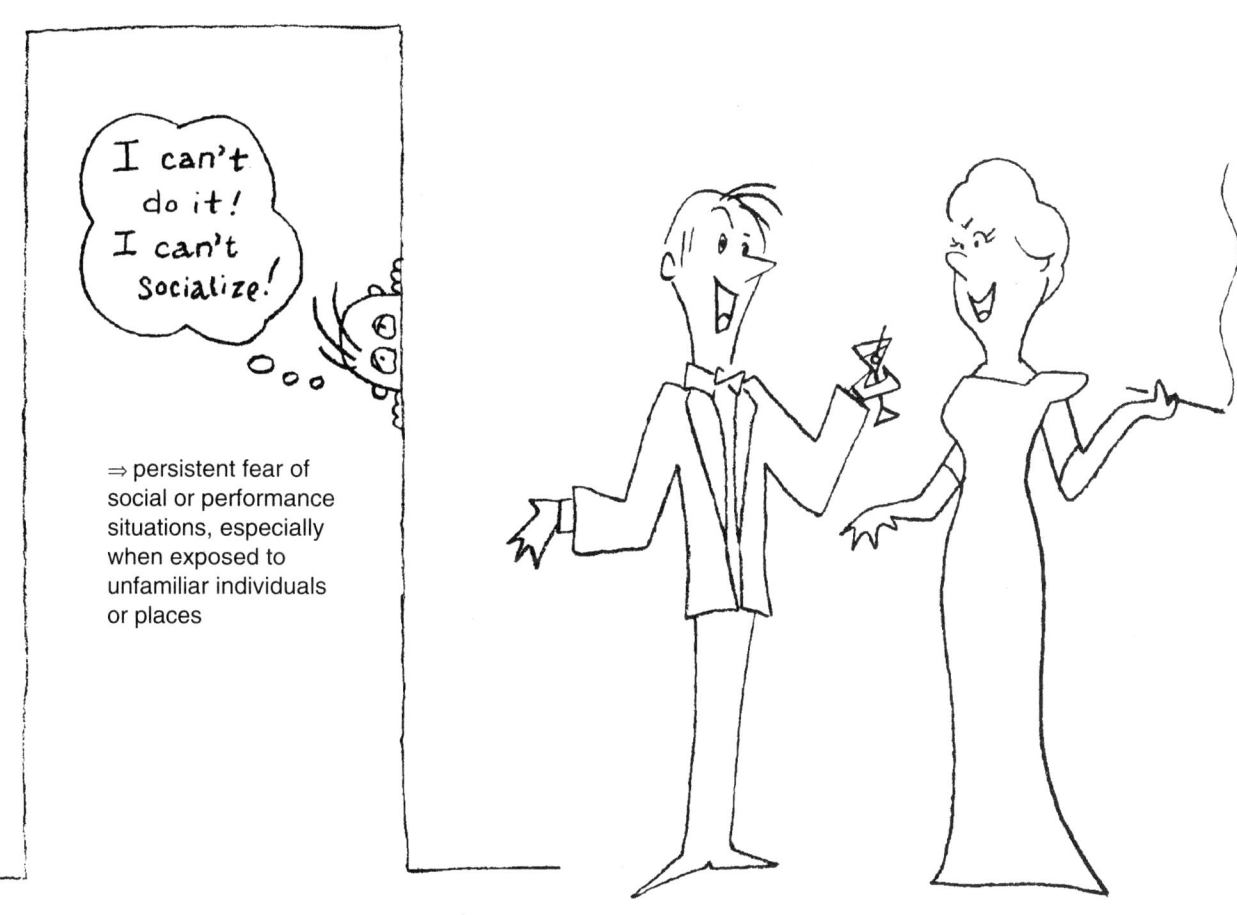

⇒ persistent fear of social or performance situations, especially when exposed to unfamiliar individuals or places

13. Disorders of Childhood and Adolescence

ATTENTION DEFICIT DISORDER (ADD, AS DEFINED BY DSM-IV-TR)

- ADD or attention deficit/hyperactivity disorder (ADHD) is characterized by symptoms being present in either an inattention or hyperactivity/impulsivity category. These symptoms are inconsistent with the child's current developmental level.

■ INATTENTION

- Often fails to give close attention to details or makes careless mistakes in schoolwork, work, or other activities
- Often has difficulty sustaining attention in tasks or play activities
- Often does not seem to listen when spoken to directly
- Often does not follow through on instructions and fails to finish schoolwork, chores, or duties in the workplace (not caused by oppositional behavior or failure to understand instructions)
- Often has difficulty organizing tasks and activities
- Often avoids, dislikes, or is reluctant to engage in tasks that require sustained mental effort (such as schoolwork or homework)
- Often loses things necessary for tasks or activities (e.g., toys, school assignments, pencils, books, or tools)
- Is often easily distracted by extraneous stimuli
- Is often forgetful in daily activities

■ HYPERACTIVITY

- Often fidgets with hands or feet or squirms in seat
- Often leaves seat in classroom or in other situations in which remaining seated is expected
- Often runs about or climbs excessively in situations in which it is inappropriate (in adolescents or adults, may be limited to subjective feelings of restlessness)
- Often has difficulty playing or engaging in leisure activities quietly
- Is often "on the go" or acts as if "driven by a motor"
- Often talks excessively

■ IMPULSIVITY

- Often blurts out answers before questions have been completed
- Often has difficulty awaiting turn
- Often interrupts or intrudes on others (e.g., butts into conversations or games)
- Symptoms must have persisted for at least 6 months. Some of these symptoms need to have been present as a child, at 7 years old or younger. The symptoms also must exist in at least two separate settings (e.g., at school and at home).

■ MISCELLANEOUS

- Affects boys more often than girls
- Approximately 10% of school-age population
- Treatment consists of stimulants, antidepressants, and α-adrenergic medications; also psychotherapy and behavior modification

Attention Deficit Disorder

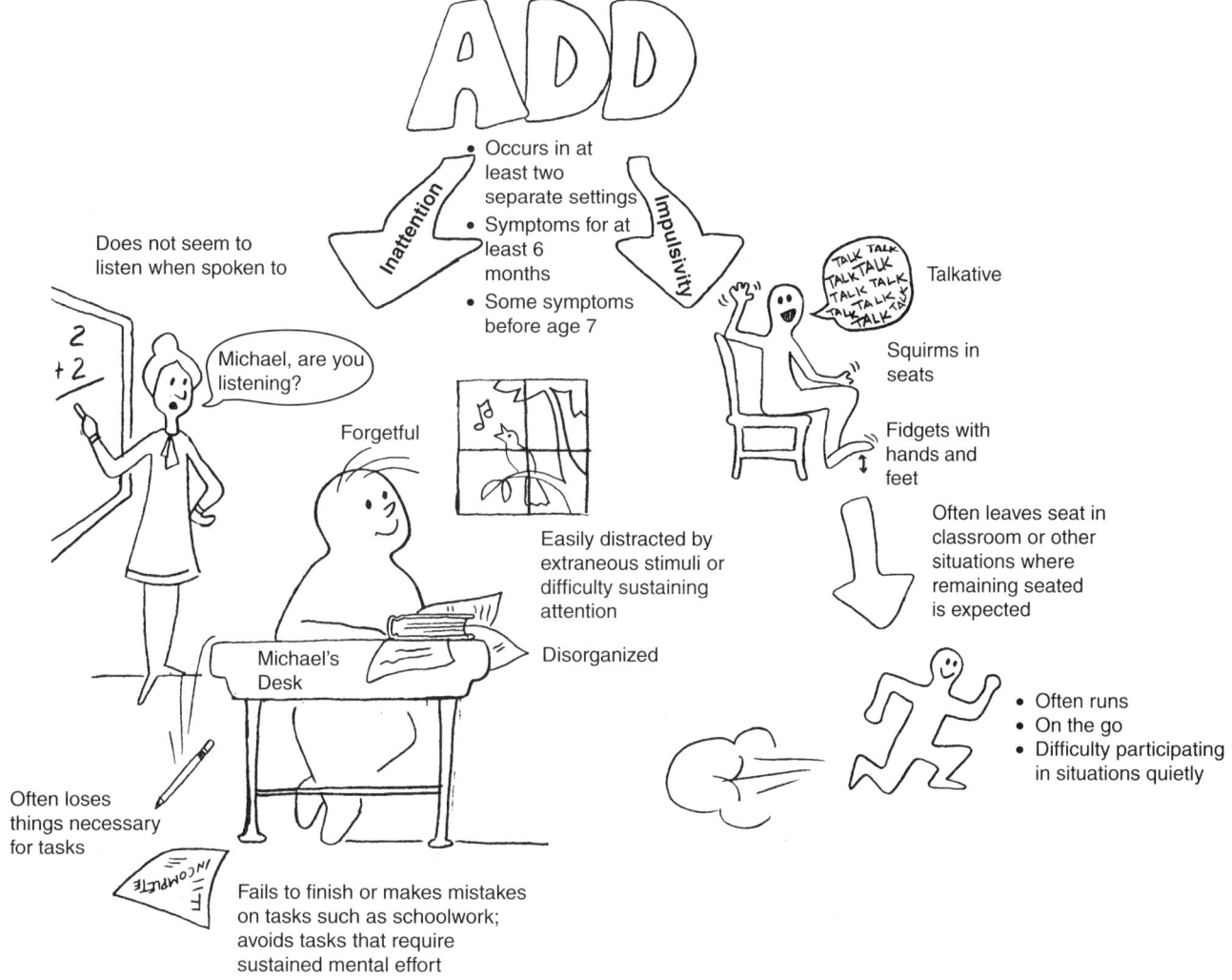

13. Disorders of Childhood and Adolescence

NOTES

TOURETTE'S DISORDER (AS DEFINED BY DSM-IV-TR)

- Both multiple motor and one or more vocal tics have been present at some time during the illness, although not necessarily concurrently. (A tic is a sudden, rapid, recurrent, nonrhythmic, stereotyped motor movement or vocalization.)
- The tics occur many times a day (usually in bouts), nearly every day or intermittently throughout a period of more than 1 year, and during this period there was never a tic-free period of more than 3 consecutive months.
- The onset is before age 18 years.
- Miscellaneous:
    o Commonly associated with attention deficit/hyperactivity disorder (ADHD) and obsessive-compulsive disorder (OCD)
    o Strong genetic component
    o Mostly affects males
    o Treatment includes neuroleptics, α-andrenergic medications, and behavioral therapy

Tourette's Disorder

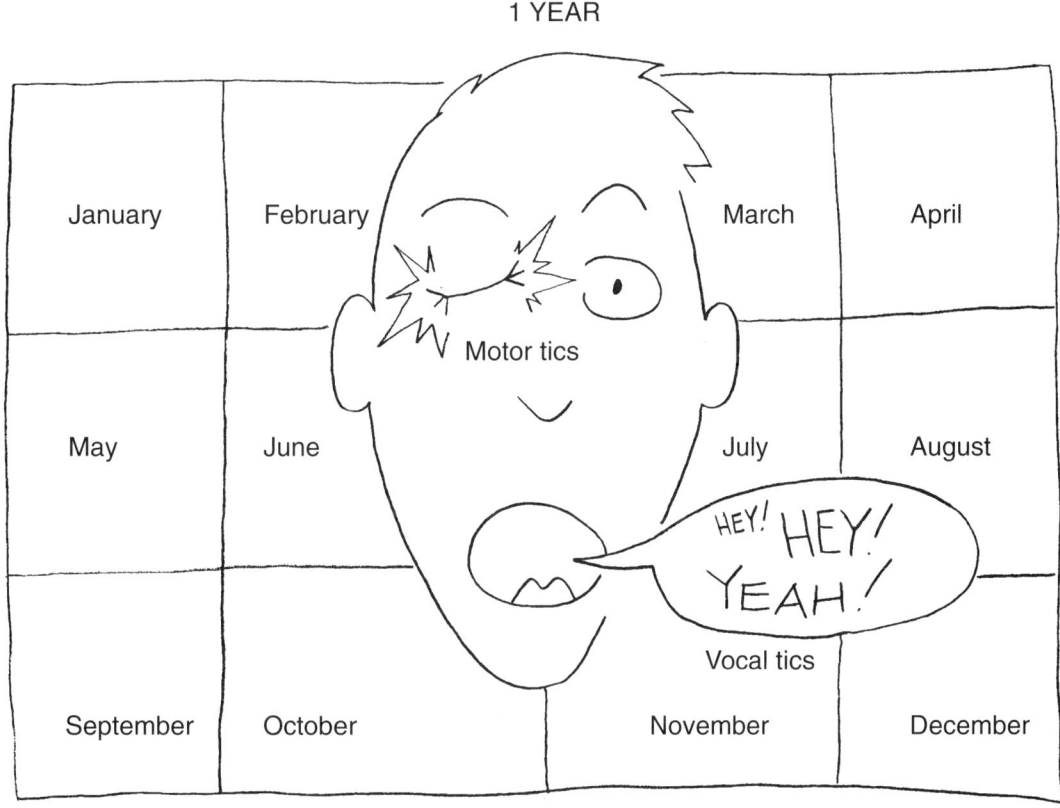

13. Disorders of Childhood and Adolescence

AUTISTIC DISORDER (AS DEFINED BY DSM-IV-TR)

A total of six (or more) items from (a), (b), and (c), with at least two from (a) and one each from (b) and (c):

(a) Qualitative impairment in social interaction, as manifested by at least two of the following:
- Marked impairment in the use of multiple nonverbal behaviors, such as eye-to-eye gaze, facial expression, body postures, and gestures to regulate social interaction
- Failure to develop peer relationships appropriate to developmental level
- Lack of spontaneous seeking to share enjoyment, interests, or achievements with other people (e.g., by a lack of showing, bringing, or pointing out objects of interest)
- Lack of social or emotional reciprocity

(b) Qualitative impairments in communication, as manifested by at least one of the following:
- Delay in, or total lack of, the development of spoken language (not accompanied by an attempt to compensate through alternative modes of communication, such as gesture or mime)
- In individuals with adequate speech, marked impairment in the ability to initiate or sustain a conversation with others
- Stereotyped and repetitive use of language or idiosyncratic language
- Lack of varied, spontaneous make-believe play or social imitative play appropriate to developmental level

(c) Restricted repetitive and stereotyped patterns of behavior, interests, and activities, as manifested by at least one of the following:
- Encompassing preoccupation with one or more stereotyped and restricted patterns of interest that is abnormal either in intensity or focus
- Apparently inflexible adherence to specific, nonfunctional routines or rituals
- Stereotyped and repetitive motor mannerisms (e.g., hand or finger flapping or twisting, or complex whole-body movements)
- Persistent preoccupation with parts of objects

Delays or abnormal functioning in at least one of the following areas, with onset before age 3 years: (1) social interaction, (2) language as used in social communication, or (3) symbolic or imaginative play.

■ MISCELLANEOUS
- Male predominance
- Strong genetic component
- Treatment: Early educational intervention; psychotherapy; behavioral therapy; medications to treat specific symptoms

Autistic Disorder

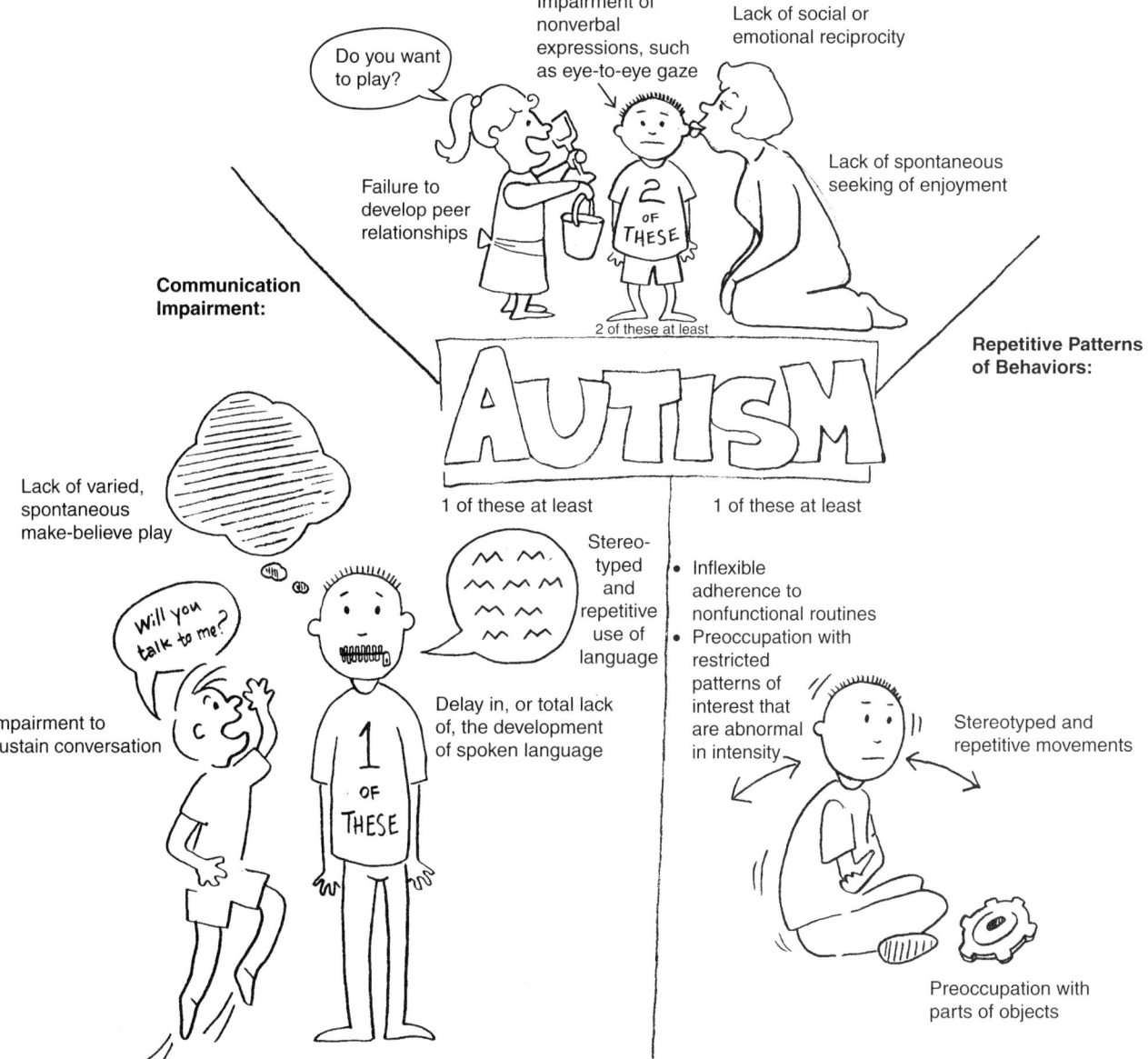

13. Disorders of Childhood and Adolescence

NOTES

ASPERGER'S DISORDER (AS DEFINED BY DSM-IV-TR)

- Qualitative impairment in social interaction, as manifested by at least two of the following:
  - Marked impairment in the use of multiple nonverbal behaviors, such as eye-to-eye gaze, facial expression, body postures, and gestures to regulate social interaction
  - Failure to develop peer relationships appropriate to developmental level
  - A lack of spontaneous seeking to share enjoyment, interests, or achievements with other people (e.g., by a lack of showing, bringing, or pointing out objects of interest to other people)
  - Lack of social or emotional reciprocity
- Restricted repetitive and stereotyped patterns of behavior, interests, and activities, as manifested by at least one of the following:
  - Encompassing preoccupation with one or more stereotyped and restricted patterns of interest that are abnormal either in intensity or focus
  - Apparently inflexible adherence to specific, nonfunctional routines or rituals
  - Stereotyped and repetitive motor mannerisms (e.g., hand or finger flapping or twisting, or complex whole-body movements)
  - Persistent preoccupation with parts of objects
- The disturbance causes clinically significant impairment in social, occupational, or other important areas of functioning.
- There is no clinically significant general delay in language (e.g., single words used by age 2 years, communicative phrases used by age 3 years).
- There is no clinically significant delay in cognitive development or in the development of age-appropriate self-help skills, adaptive behavior (other than in social interaction), and curiosity about the environment in childhood.

Asperger's Disorder

Asperger's is similar to autism in social interaction impairment and repetitive patterns of behavior, BUT with no communication/language delays!

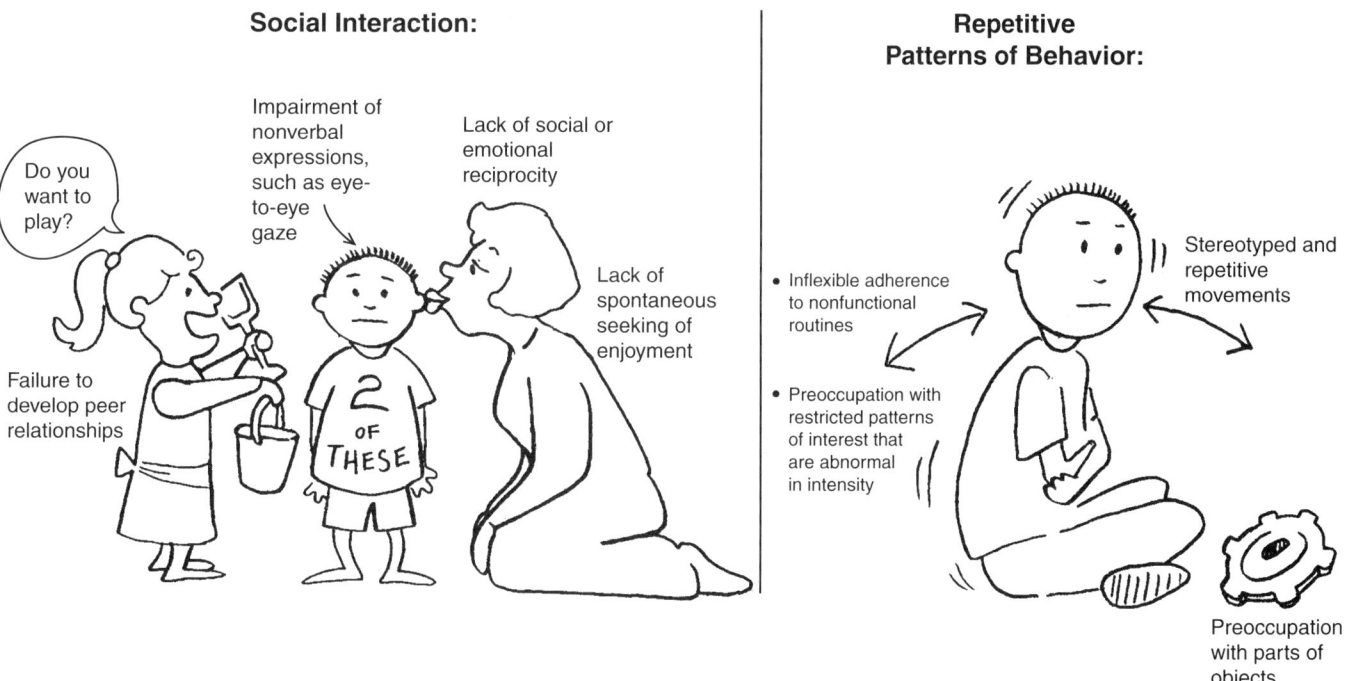

13. Disorders of Childhood and Adolescence

RETT'S DISORDER (AS DEFINED BY DSM-IV-TR)

- A period of normal prenatal and perinatal development until 5 months of age, at which time all of the following occurs:
  - Deceleration in growth of head circumference between ages 5 and 48 months
  - Between the ages of 5 and 30 months, loss of purposeful movements of hands and replaced by stereotyped hand movements (e.g., hand wringing)
  - Loss of social interaction
  - Incoordinated gait or trunk movements
  - Severe impairment of language skills and severe psychomotor retardation
- There is a prevalence of the disease in girls, and the etiology is a mutation in the MECP2 gene

Rett's Disorder

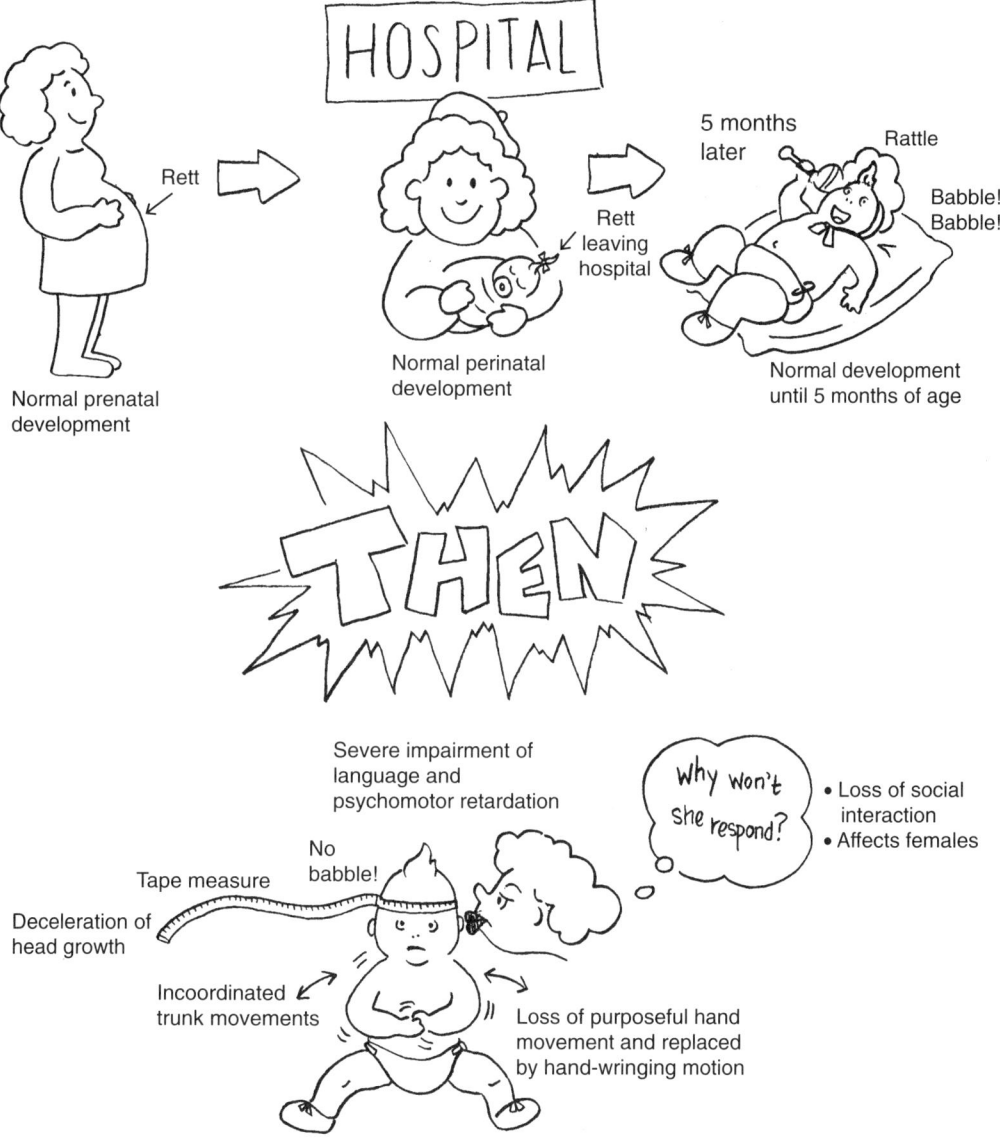

13. Disorders of Childhood and Adolescence

OPPOSITIONAL DEFIANT DISORDER (AS DEFINED BY DSM-IV-TR)

- A pattern of negativistic, hostile, and defiant behavior lasting at least 6 months, during which four (or more) of the following are present:
    - Often loses temper
    - Often argues with adults
    - Often actively defies or refuses to comply with adults' requests or rules
    - Often deliberately annoys people
    - Often blames others for his or her mistakes or misbehavior
    - Is often touchy or easily annoyed by others
    - Is often angry and resentful
    - Is often spiteful or vindictive
- Treatment: Usually behavioral therapy, implemented through parent training

Oppositional Defiant Disorder

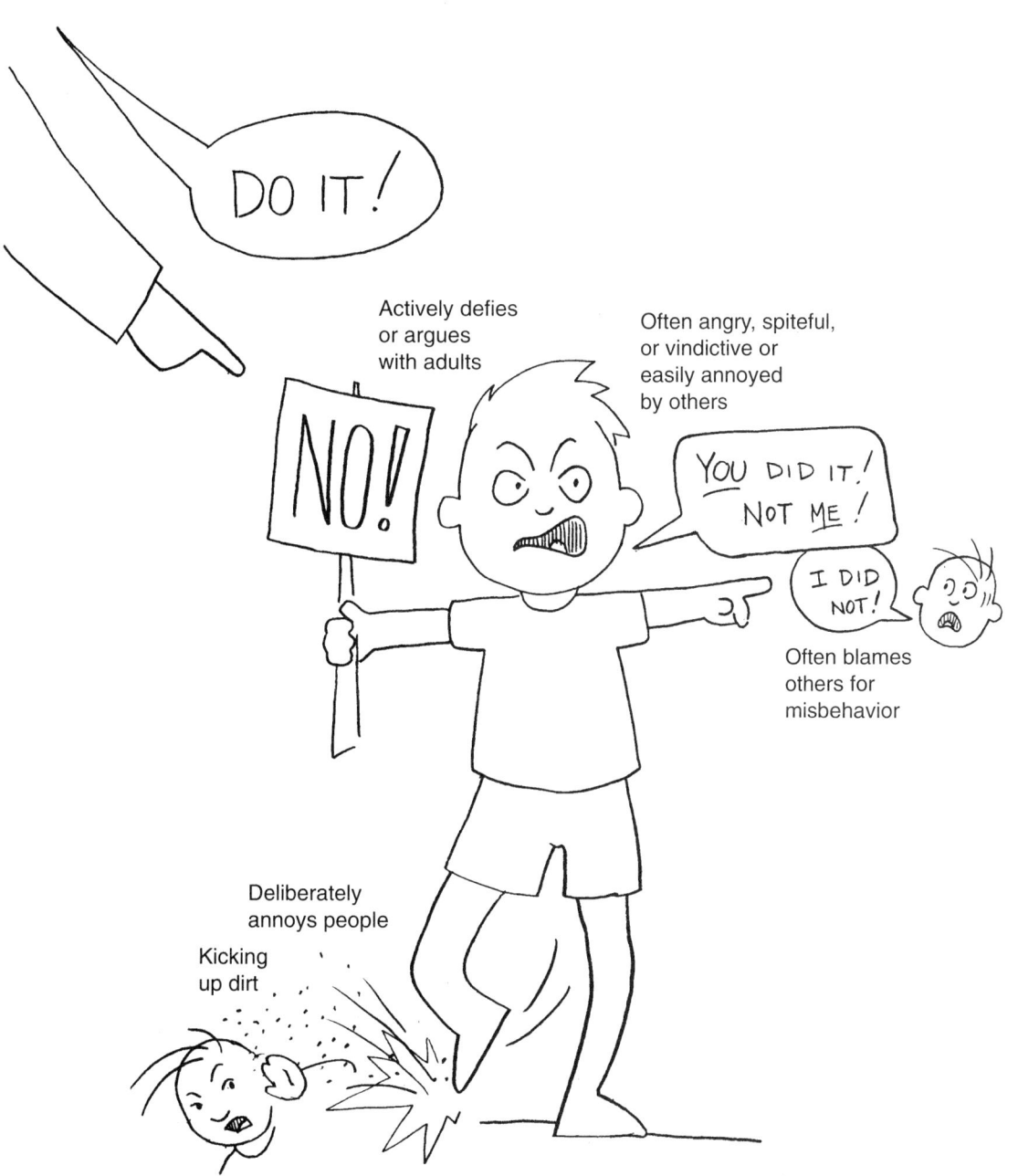

13. Disorders of Childhood and Adolescence

NOTES

CONDUCT DISORDER (AS DEFINED BY DSM-IV-TR)

A repetitive and persistent pattern of behavior in which the basic rights of others or major age-appropriate societal norms or rules are violated, as manifested by the presence of three (or more) of the following criteria in the past 12 months, with at least one criterion present in the past 6 months:

- **Aggression to people and animals**
    - Often bullies, threatens, or intimidates others
    - Often initiates physical fights
    - Has used a weapon that can cause serious physical harm to others (e.g., a bat, brick, broken bottle, knife, gun)
    - Has been physically cruel to people
    - Has been physically cruel to animals
    - Has stolen while confronting a victim (e.g., mugging, purse snatching, extortion, armed robbery)
    - Has forced someone into sexual activity
- **Destruction of property**
    - Has deliberately engaged in fire setting with the intention of causing serious damage
    - Has deliberately destroyed others' property (other than by fire setting)
- **Deceitfulness or theft**
    - Has broken into someone's house, building, or car
    - Often lies to obtain goods or favors or to avoid obligations (i.e., "cons" others)
    - Has stolen items of nontrivial value without confronting a victim (e.g., shoplifting, but without breaking and entering; forgery)
- **Serious violations of rules**
    - Often stays out at night despite parental prohibitions, beginning before age 13 years
    - Has run away from home overnight at least twice while living in parental or parental surrogate home (or once without returning for a lengthy period)
    - Is often truant from school, beginning before age 13 years

If the individual is age 18 years or older, criteria are not met for Antisocial Personality Disorder.

Conduct Disorder

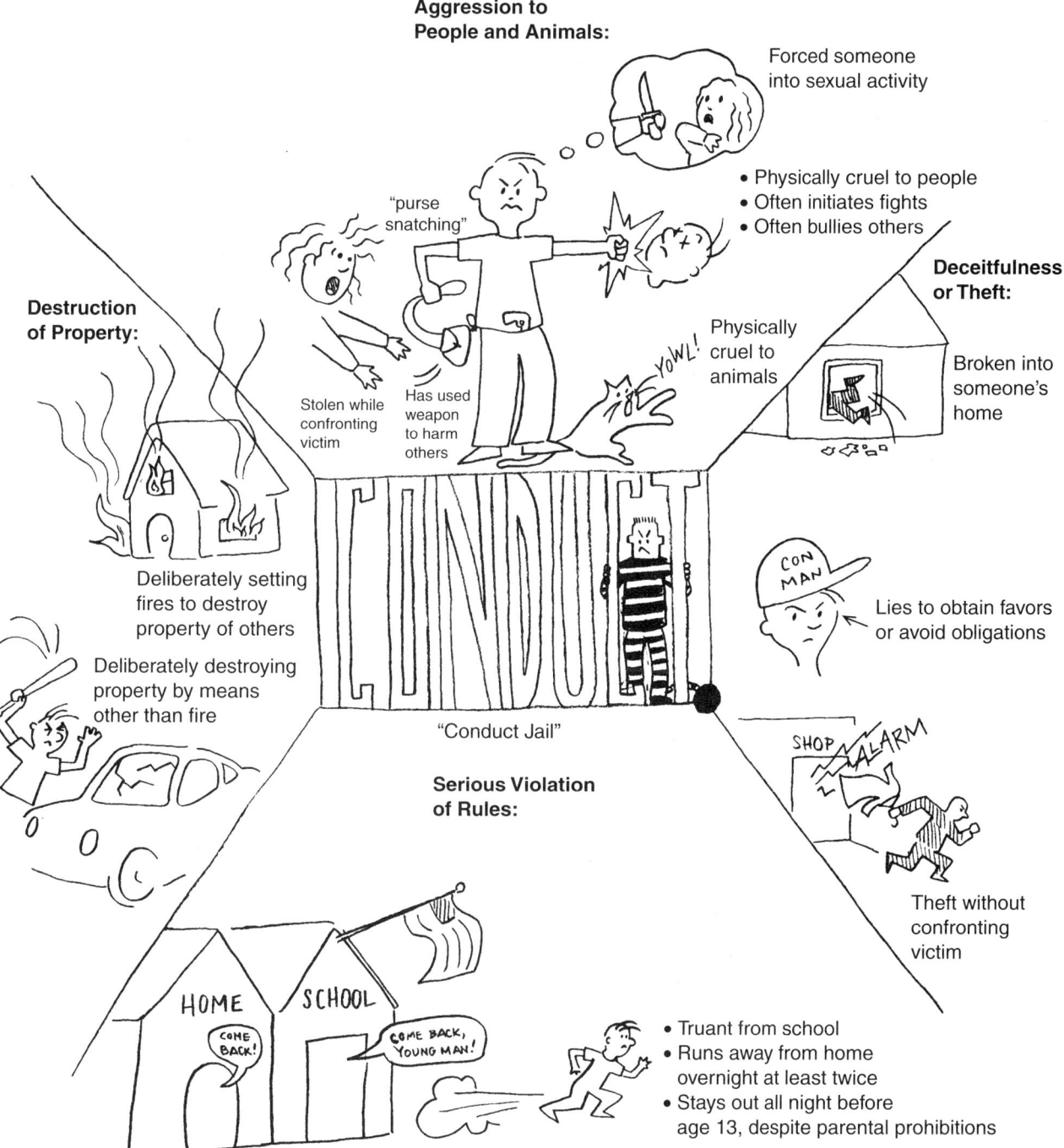

14. Psychotherapies

NOTES

PSYCHOANALYSIS

The goal of psychoanalysis is to reveal repressed emotions or experiences from the unconscious and allow them to develop into the personality of the patient.

- **Free Association**
  - The patient is instructed to say whatever comes to mind to reveal unconscious experiences
    ⇒ "Free your mind!"
- **Dream Interpretation**
  - The patient's dreams are openly discussed to reveal unconscious fears or hopes
    ⇒ Dream on a cloud
- **Transference Analysis**
  - The patient's relationship with the therapist is examined to reveal unconscious emotions from past relationships

Psychoanalysis

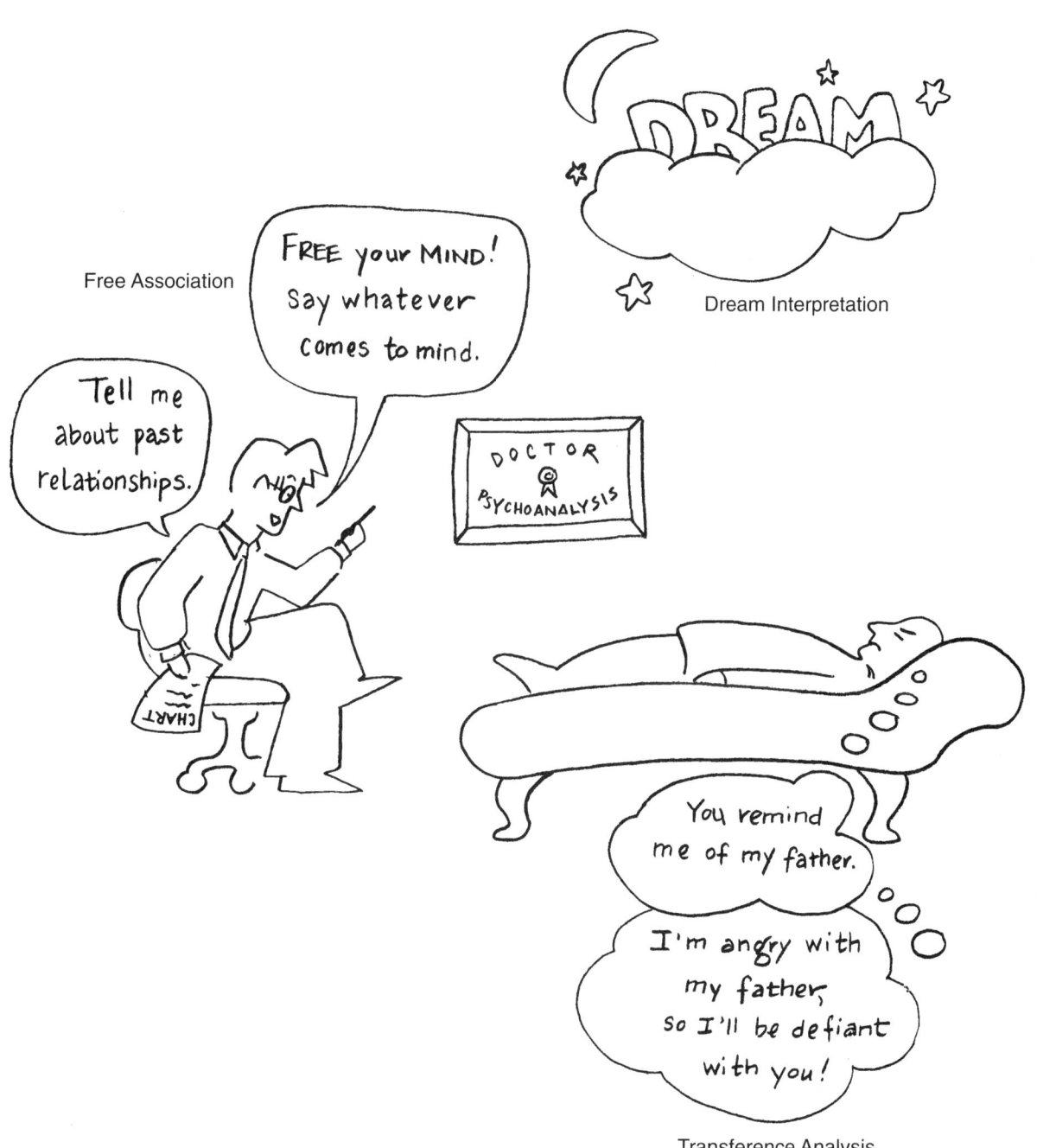

14. Psychotherapies

NOTES

BEHAVIORAL THEORY

- **Modeling**
    - Learning by imitating actions of others
        - ⇒ woman imitating other woman
- **Classical Conditioning**
    - Learning by pairing different stimuli to achieve the desired response
        - ⇒ "I'm not scared of this picture of a plane. Now, I'm not scared of planes!"
- **Operant Conditioning**
    - Influences allow for learning new behaviors and terminating old, unwanted behaviors
        - ⇒ woman smashing old behaviors

Behavioral Theory

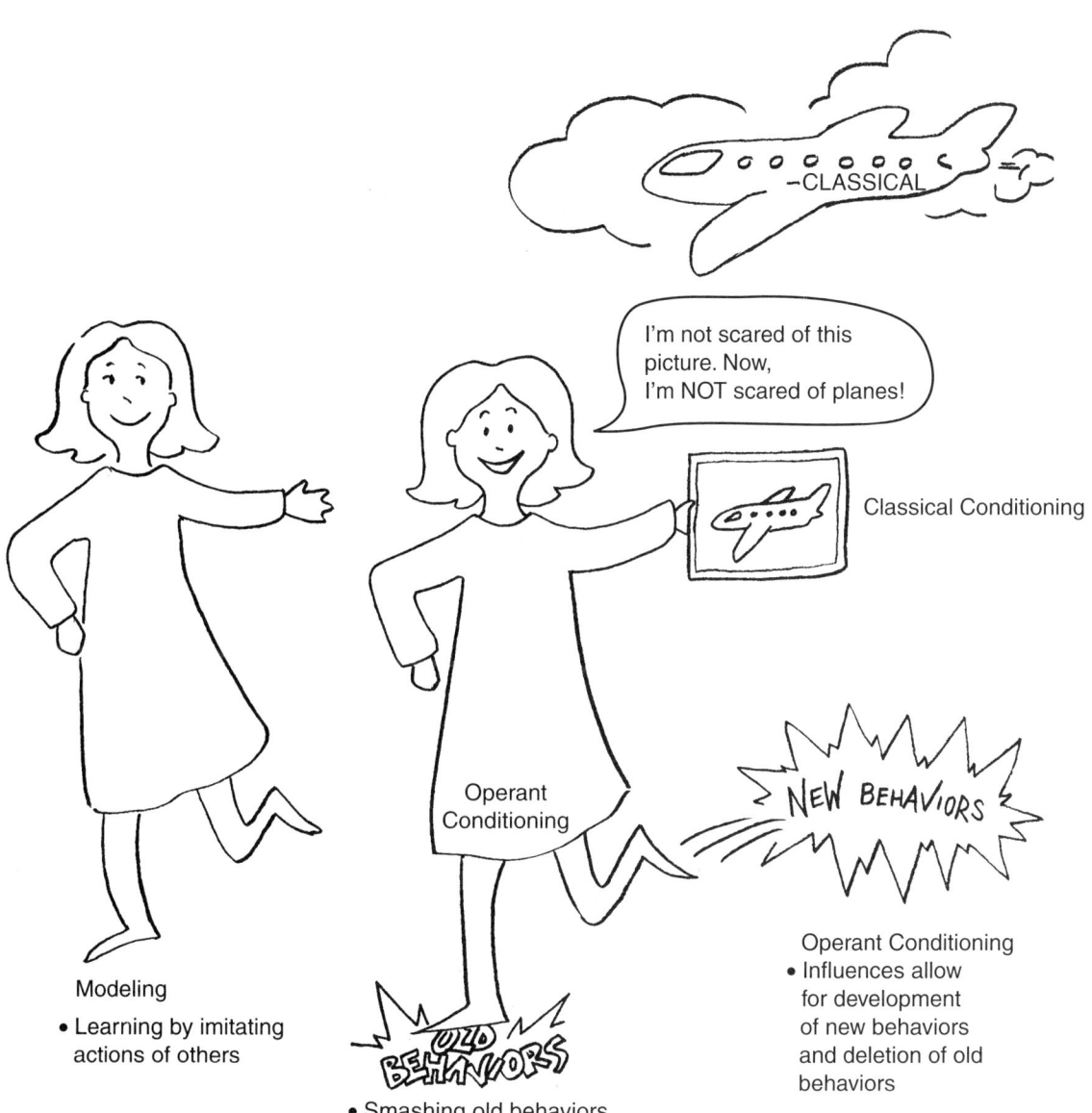

14. Psychotherapies

BEHAVIORAL AND COGNITIVE THERAPIES

- **Systemic Desensitization**
  - For the treatment of phobias
  - Patient is repeatedly exposed to objects related to fear and taught to simultaneously relax
    - ⇒ Patients who are scared of flying are exposed to pictures of planes and toy planes and taught to relax, so they will eventually respond the same with an actual flight
- **Aversive Conditioning**
  - ⇒ shock
  - Painful stimulus is paired with unwanted behavior
    - ⇒ Patients receive a shock with smoking, so they will associate smoking with pain and quit smoking
- **Implosion**
  - Patients repeatedly imagine feared experience to eventually overcome fear
- **Flooding**
  - Patients are exposed directly to the actual fear
- **Cognitive Therapy**
  - Patients replace negative feelings with positive feelings about self
    - ⇒ "I am beautiful! I am smart! I am successful!"
- **Token Therapy**
  - ⇒ token = coins
  - Patients are given a reward to reinforce proper behavior
  - Patients then perform proper behavior without reinforcement

Behavioral and Cognitive Therapies

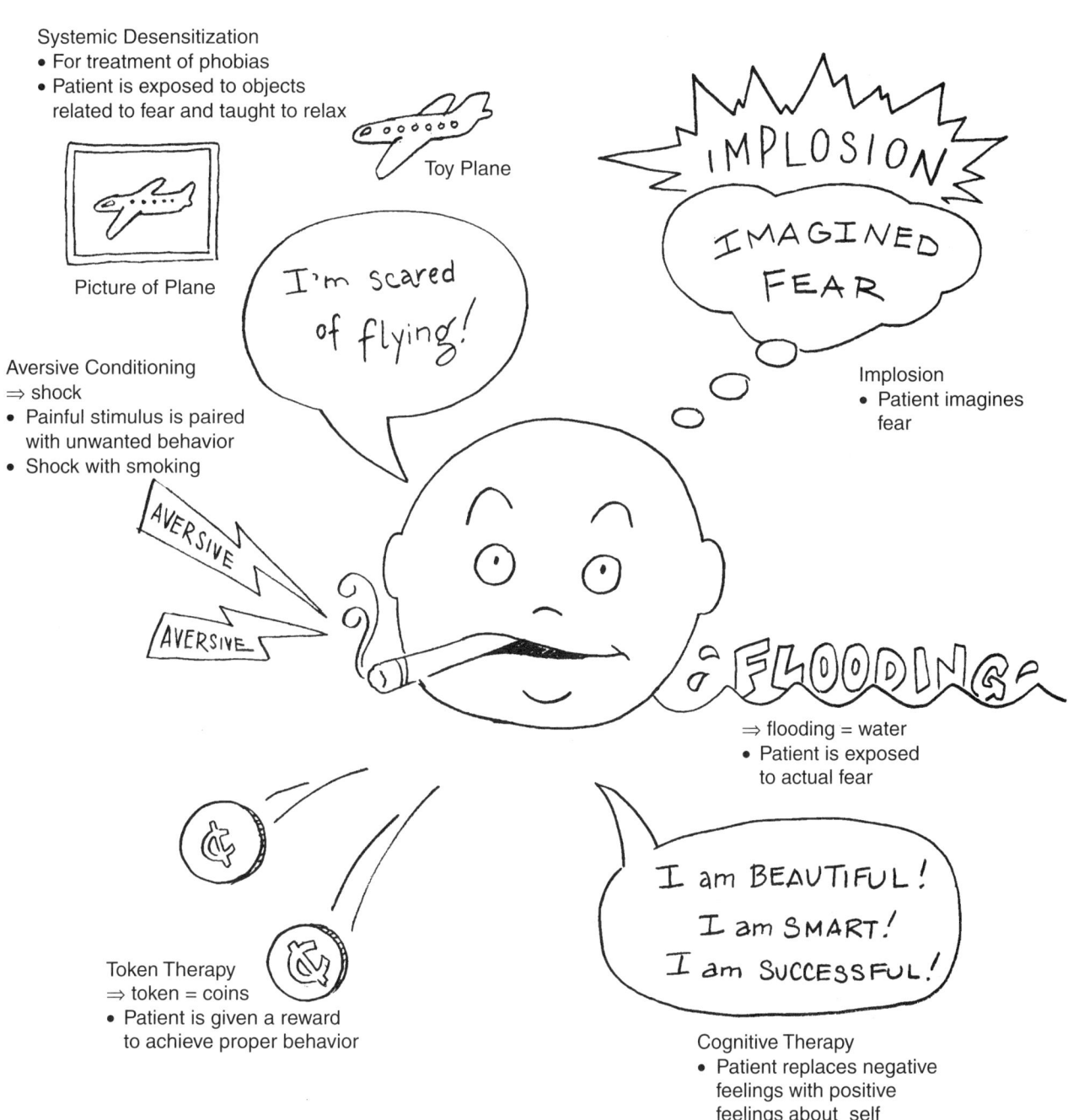

15. Sleep and Sleep Disorders

STAGES OF SLEEP

- NREM Sleep – Nonrapid eye movement; non-REM
  - Stage 0: Awake; alpha rhythm
  - Stage 1: Transition from wakefulness to sleep; light sleep
  - Stage 2: Transition between delta and REM sleep; medium sleep; sleep spindles and K complexes
- Delta Sleep – non-REM
  - Slow-wave sleep
  - Stage 3: Deeper depth of sleep than stage 2; approximately 20% to 50% of a period consists of delta waves
  - Stage 4: Greater delta-wave activity than stage 3; very deep sleep; greater than 50% of a period consists of delta waves
- REM Sleep – Rapid eye movement
  - Active EEG
  - Dream sleep
  - Depth of sleep between stage 2 and stage 3
  - Loss of muscle tone except ocular and respiratory muscles
  - REM sleep occurs 60 to 90 minutes after onset of sleep
- Polysomnography is used to determine sleep states and includes electroencephalograms (EEGs), electromyograms (EMGs), electrocardiograms (ECGs), and eye movements.
- Normal sleep progresses through the four stages of non-REM sleep in order 1 through 4. Stage 2 then occurs as a transition between delta sleep and REM sleep. REM sleep occurs next, and the entire cycle lasts about 90 minutes. Four to six cycles occur each night in a normal adult.

Stages of Sleep

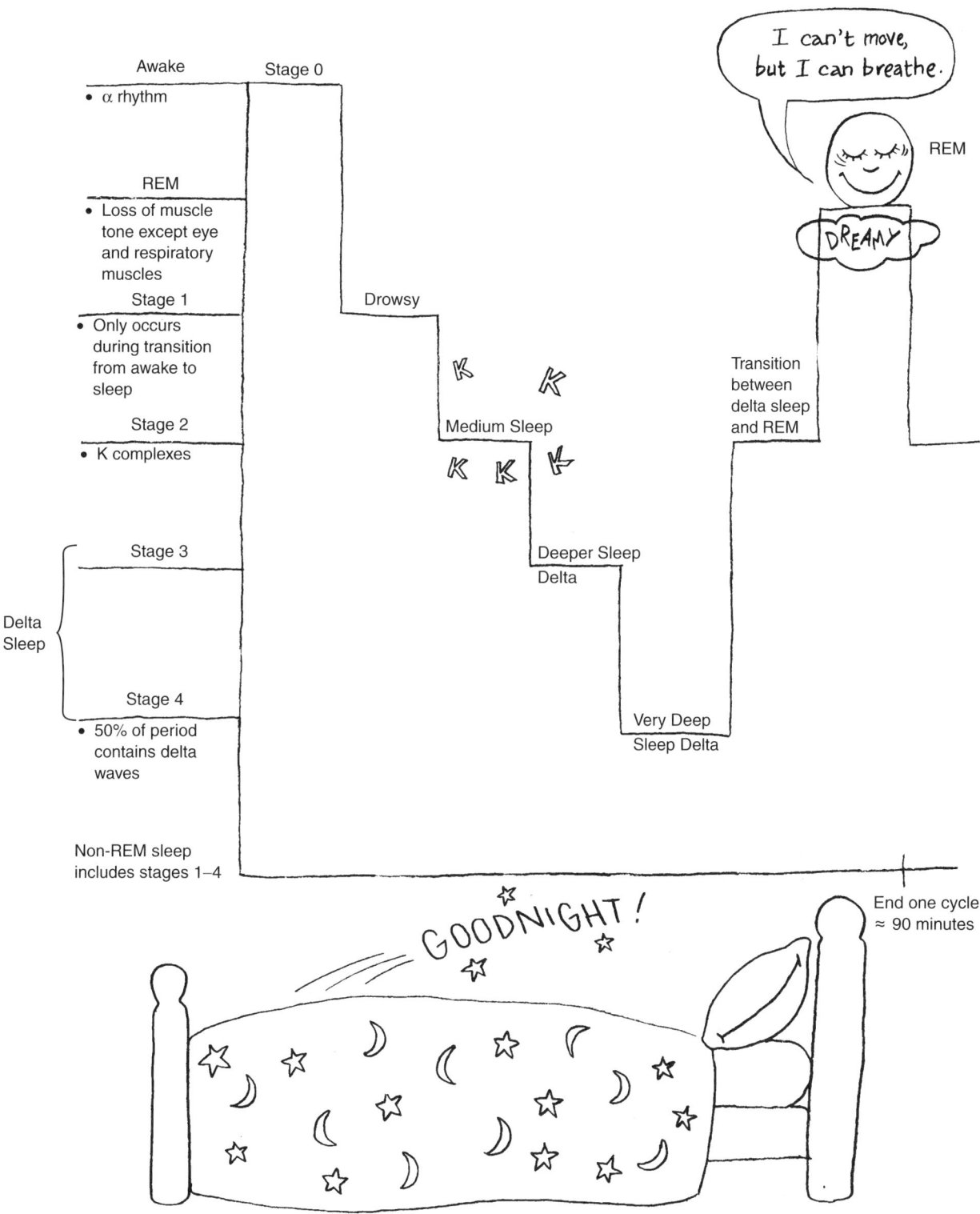

15. Sleep and Sleep Disorders

SLEEP DISORDERS: DYSSOMNIAS

Dyssomnias include five primary sleep disorders consisting of difficulty initiating and maintaining sleep and excessive sleep. According to DSM-IV-TR criteria, all of the disorders cause distress or affect social functioning or work and are not caused by a physical or mental condition, medications, or substance abuse.

■ PRIMARY INSOMNIA

- DSM-IV-TR criteria include difficulty falling asleep or maintaining sleep
- Anxiety and depression often coexist
- Treatment includes Zolpidem (Ambien) and Zaleplon (Sonata), which are both benzodiazepine agonists. Short-acting benzodiazopines may be used temporarily. Sedating antidepressants such as trazodone (Desyrel) and amitriptyline (Elavil) may also be used
  Zolpidem ⇒ pie
- Also advise proper sleep techniques:
  o Discontinue caffeine, nicotine, and alcohol
    ⇒ cigarettes, soda, beer in trash
  o Avoid daytime napping
  o Avoid exercise before sleeping, but encourage regular exercise
  o Avoid meals before sleeping
  o Keep a consistent schedule of waking and sleeping at the same time every day
    ⇒ alarm clock

■ PRIMARY HYPERSOMNIA

- DSM-IV-TR criteria include:
  o Excessive sleepiness occurring for one month
  o Associated with daytime sleepiness
- Treatment includes stimulants for daytime sleepiness

■ NARCOLEPSY

- DSM-IV-TR criteria include:
  o Sleep attacks during the day with abnormal REM sleep (e.g., sleep paralysis, sleep-onset REM, cataplexy, hallucinations)
    ⇒ sun with REM
- Cataplexy involves the sudden onset of sleep with reversible bilateral loss of skeletal muscle tone and may be triggered by emotions
    cataplexy ⇒ sleeping cat
- Hypnagogic hallucinations occur at the beginning of sleep
- May be familial, and greater than 90% have HLA-DR2
- Daytime naps often relieve sleepiness
- Treatment includes Modanfinil, a nonamphetamine stimulant approved for narcolepsy. Methylphenidate (Ritalin), a stimulant, is also used.
    Ritalin ⇒ fin

■ BREATHING-RELATED SLEEP DISORDER (SLEEP APNEA)

- DSM-IV-TR criteria include sleep disruption resulting in daytime sleepiness
- Sleep apnea involves abnormal breathing, snoring, frequent awakenings, and oxygen desaturation
- Sleep apnea can result in depression, anxiety, and memory and concentration disturbances
- Central sleep apnea is caused by brainstem dysfunction
    ⇒ flower stem on brain
- Obstructive sleep apnea is caused by airway obstruction
    ⇒ X on neck
- Treatment includes continuous positive airway pressure (CPAP)
- Weight loss or nasal surgery may also be indicated

■ CIRCADIAN RHYTHM SLEEP DISORDER

    ⇒ clock
- DSM-IV-TR criteria include mismatch between intrinsic circadian rhythm and actual sleep periods
- May occur with jet lag, long work shifts, or night shifts
    ⇒ jet

Dyssomnias

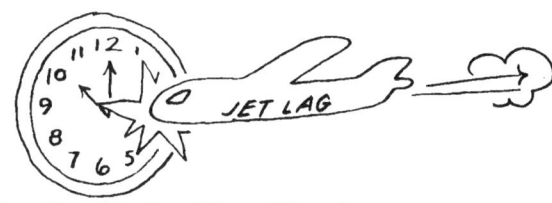

Circadian Rhythm Sleep Disorder
⇒ clock
- Mismatch between circadian rhythm and actual sleep periods
- Occurs with jet lag and long shifts
  ⇒ jet

Sleep Apnea
- Involves snoring, frequent awakenings, and O_2 desaturation
- Central sleep apnea is caused by a brainstem dysfunction
  ⇒ flower stem on brain
- Obstructive sleep apnea
  ⇒ X on neck
- Treatment includes CPAP and weight loss

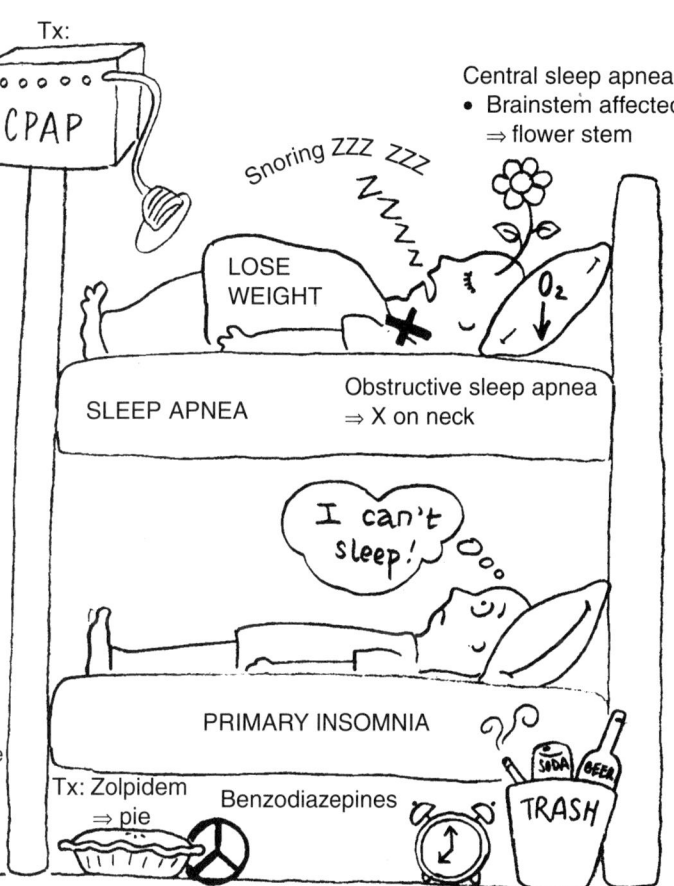

Central sleep apnea
- Brainstem affected
  ⇒ flower stem

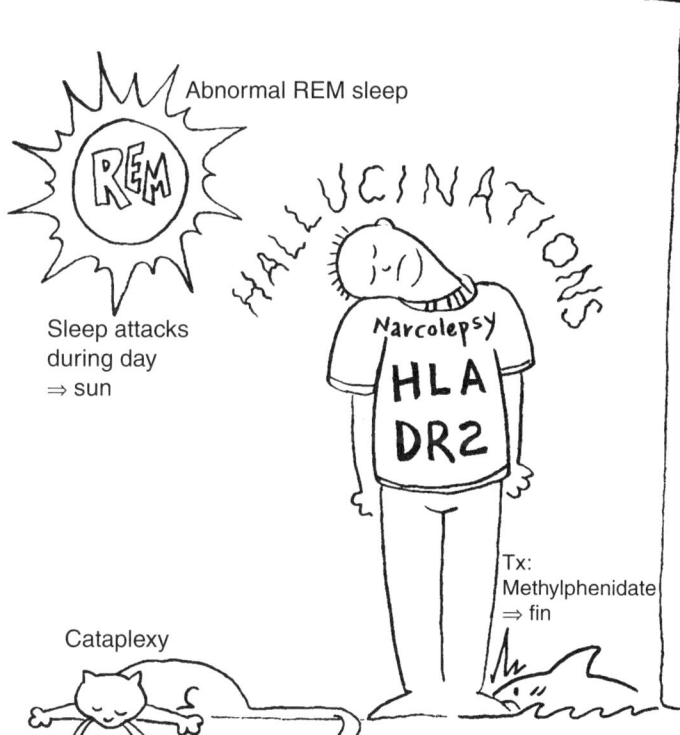

Narcolepsy
- Sleep attacks during the day with abnormal REM sleep
  ⇒ sun with REM
- Cataplexy ⇒ sleeping cat
  - Sudden onset of sleep
  - Reversible bilateral loss of skeletal muscle tone
- HLA-DR2 in 90%
- Hypnagogic hallucinations
- Treatment includes stimulants such as methylphenidate (Ritalin)
  ⇒ fin

Primary Insomnia
- Difficulty falling asleep or maintaining sleep
- Treatment includes:
  - Zolpidem (Ambien) ⇒ pie
  - Short-acting benzodiazepines
  - Sedating antidepressants (trazodone or amitriptyline)
- Proper sleep techniques
  - Avoid caffeine, nicotine, and alcohol
    ⇒ cigarettes, soda, and beer in trash
  - Avoid daytime napping
  - Avoid meals before sleeping
  - Keep a consistent schedule
    ⇒ alarm clock

15. Sleep and Sleep Disorders

NOTES

SLEEP DISORDERS: PARASOMNIAS

⇒ Parasomnias = Pair of Pears
- Parasomnias include three primary sleep disorders and involve behavioral events that occur during sleep:

■ SLEEPWALKING DISORDER

- Walking during sleep initiated during slow-wave (delta) sleep
    ⇒ slow-wave sleep = walking on wave
- Accompanied by confusion and complex behaviors and motor activity

■ NIGHTMARE DISORDER

- Scary dreams that occur during REM sleep and usually wake a person from sleep
    ⇒ bad dream
    ⇒ awaken from sleep = eyes open

■ SLEEP TERROR DISORDER

- Sudden episodes of apparent terror during slow-wave (delta) sleep. May scream or cry out, but do not usually awaken during the episode
    ⇒ slow-wave sleep = walking on wave
    ⇒ do not awaken = eyes closed

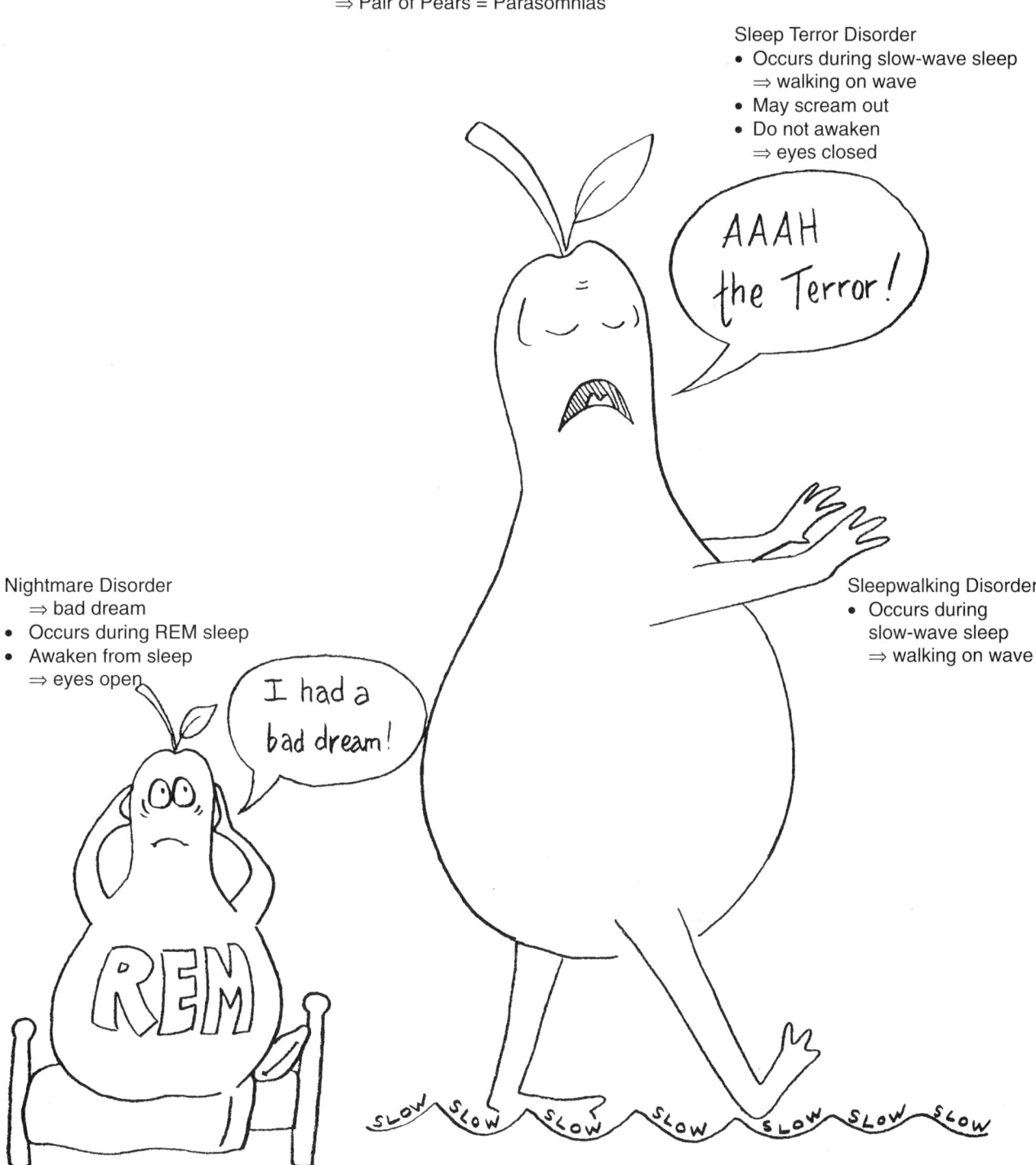

16. Ego Defenses

EGO DEFENSES

Ego defense mechanisms are used by the ego to protect self-esteem, decrease anxiety, and avoid conflict.

- **Repression**
  - The fundamental defense mechanism
  - Unacceptable feelings are sent to the unconscious
    - ⇒ Bring feelings to the Unconscious Store
    - ⇒ "Don't Remember" at the Unconscious Store

The following are mature defense mechanisms:

- **Altruism:** Helping others to avoid unacceptable personal feelings
  - ⇒ Woman feeling guilty gives money to charity
- **Humor:** Uncomfortable feelings are expressed in a humorous way
  - ⇒ Bald man makes jokes about buying a clown wig
- **Sublimation:** Changes unacceptable feelings to be more socially acceptable
  - ⇒ Man kicks ugly feelings to change them into pretty feelings
- **Suppression:** Unacceptable emotions are not dealt with by the individual
  - ⇒ "I'm not dealing with my emotions!"

Altruism, Repression, Humor, Sublimation, Suppression

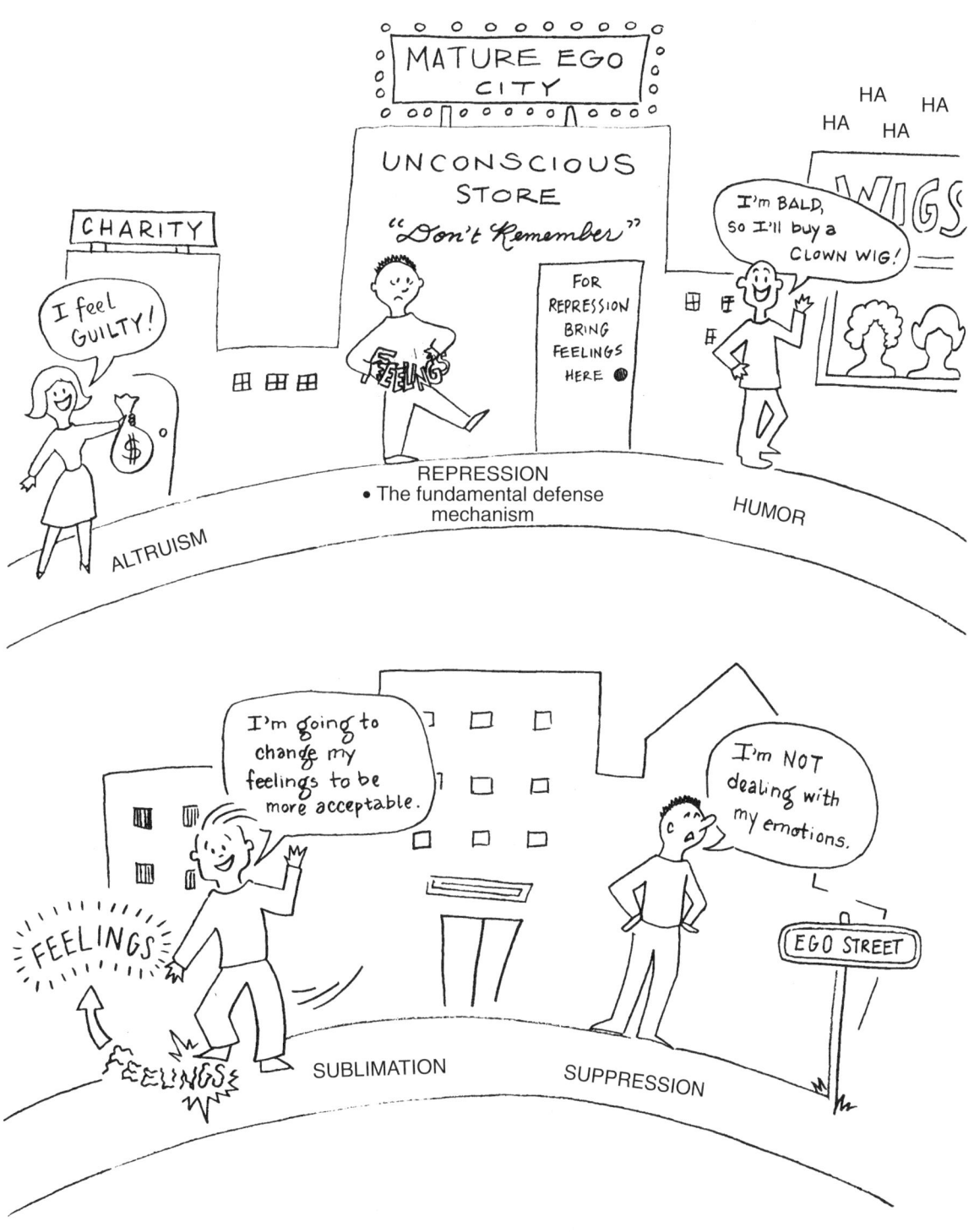

16. Ego Defenses

NOTES

MORE EGO DEFENSES

- **Acting Out:** Behaving in an unacceptable manner to avoid emotions and gain attention
    ⇒ Good girl steals clothing from the Acting Out Store
- **Splitting:** Separates people into two opposite categories (e.g., good or bad)
    ⇒ Good or Bad Store is split in two
- **Regression:** Converting back to youthful behavior; often seen with Dependent Personality Disorder
    ⇒ Adult man wants his mommy
- **Denial:** Refusing to accept reality despite definitive evidence
    ⇒ Woman insists test results are wrong at the Denial Clinic
- **Rationalization:** Converting an unacceptable outcome into a reasonable explanation
    ⇒ Girl is now glad she did not make the cheerleading squad because she now believes cheerleading is stupid
- **Reaction Formation:** Avoiding unacceptable feelings by converting them into the opposite
    ⇒ Woman who hates her boss tells her boss, "You're great!"

Acting Out, Splitting, Regression, Denial, Rationalization, Reaction Formation

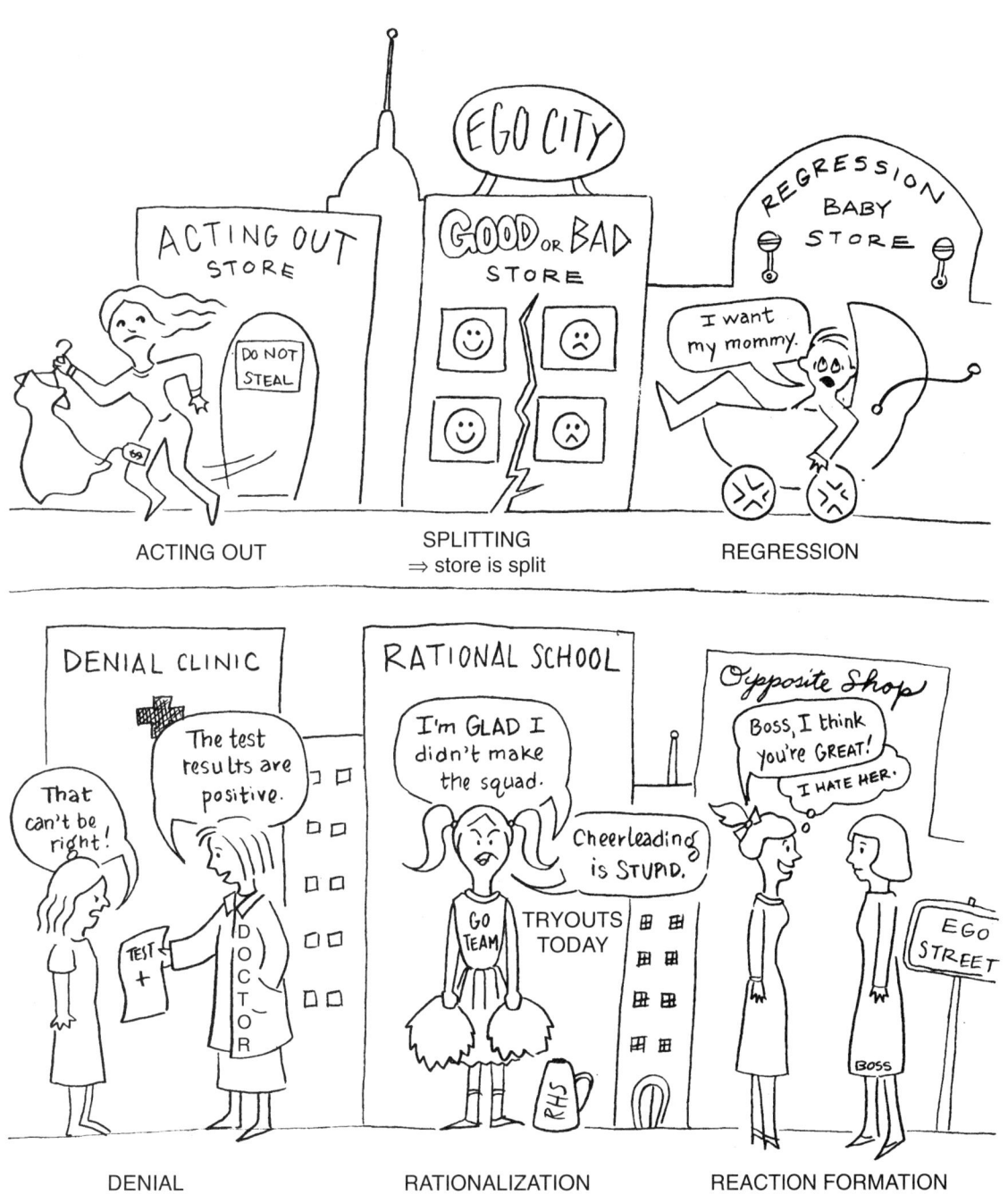

16. Ego Defenses

NOTES

EVEN MORE EGO DEFENSES

- **Projection:** Unacceptable feelings are attributed to others
    - ⇒ Woman who believes all men are bad also thinks her husband is cheating on her
- **Displacement:** Negative feelings are redirected to create a more tolerable emotion
    - ⇒ Boss who is mad at his wife later yells at a female co-worker
- **Identification:** Behaving like someone else
    - ⇒ Father yells at his son because his father yelled at him when he was young
- **Intellectualization:** Avoidance by expressing emotions in a more complicated manner
    - ⇒ Computer man avoids emotion by using his brain
- **Dissociation:** Separate one's self from emotions and others
    - ⇒ Man separating emotions from himself
    - ⇒ "Everyone stay away!"
- **Undoing:** Reversing wrong behavior by implementing right behavior
    - ⇒ Woman magically reverses wrong by doing right at the Undo It Magic Shop

Projection, Displacement, Identification, Intellectualization, Dissociation, Undoing

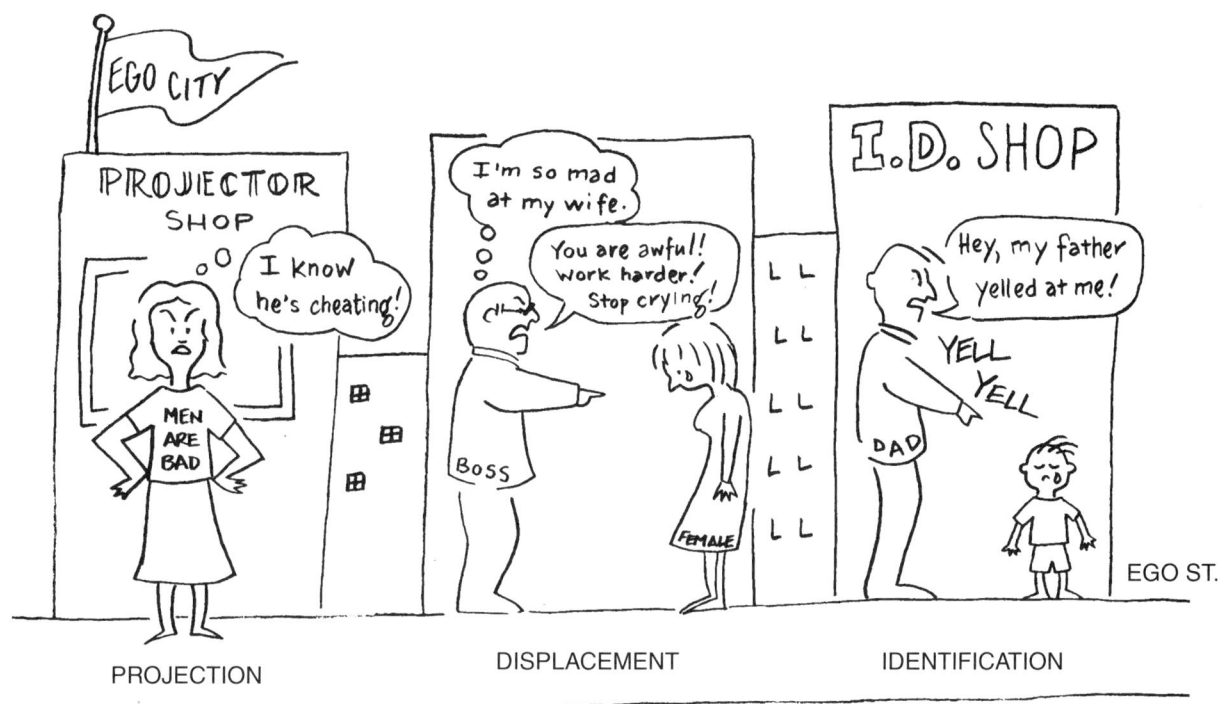

PROJECTION

DISPLACEMENT

IDENTIFICATION

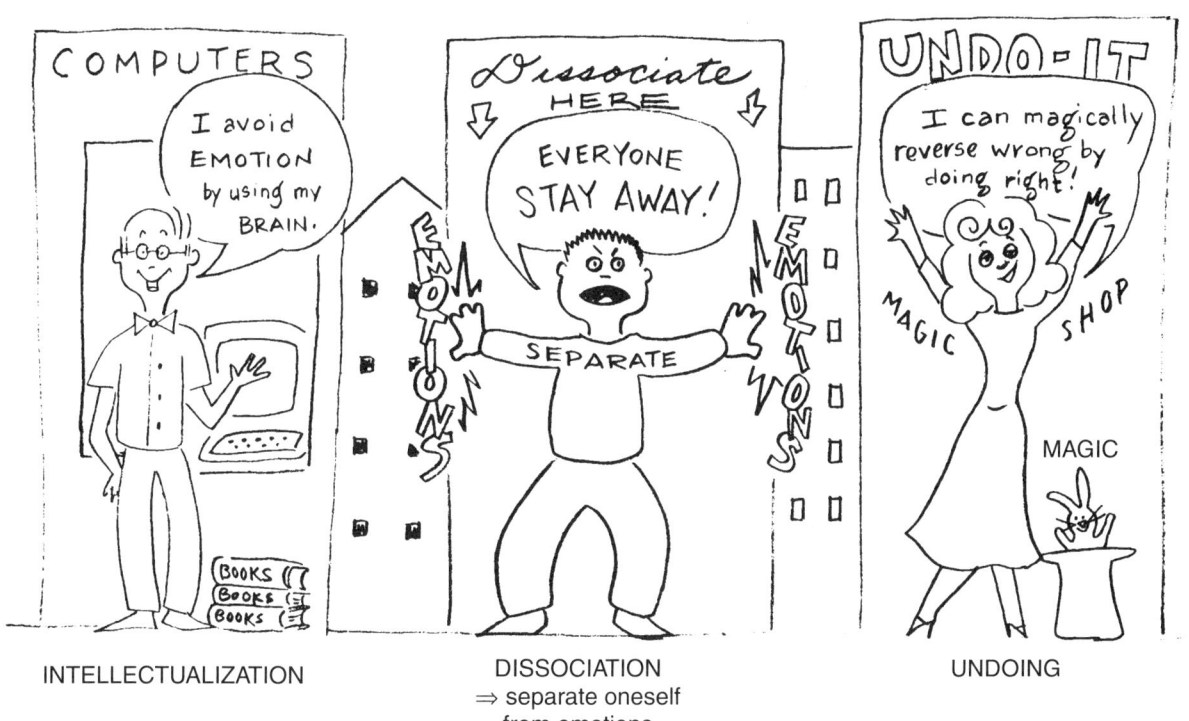

INTELLECTUALIZATION

DISSOCIATION
⇒ separate oneself from emotions

UNDOING

Appendices

APPENDIX A

■ TERMS TO UNDERSTAND AND REMEMBER

- **Illusion:** misinterpretation of sensory perceptions
- **Delusion:** fixed and false belief inconsistent with individual's experience and environment; has no basis in reality
- **Hallucination:** false perceptions of the senses (visual, auditory, or olfactory) that are inconsistent with any external stimuli
- **Judgment:** ability to understand relationships between facts and draw proper conclusions
- **Insight:** ability of the patient to understand his or her disease process and realize the need for treatment
- **Thought process:** how thoughts are connected or associated with one another
- **Thought content:** types of thoughts that an individual has
- **Affect:** emotional response to experience; described as appropriate, inappropriate, flat, blunted, labile, full, or constricted
- **Mood:** steady or sustained emotional state, such as happy or depressed
- **Broadcasting:** others can hear an individual's thoughts
- **Thought insertion:** thoughts are being inserted into individual's mind by external means
- **Ideas of reference:** type of delusion; individual believes an event is exclusively connected to him or her (e.g., person believes statement on TV or radio has special reference to him or her)
- **Blocking:** abrupt cessation of communication before discussion is finished
- **Neologisms:** made-up words that are meaningful only to patient
- **Flight of ideas:** thoughts proceeding at such a rapid pace that patient is unable to communicate them
- **Derealization:** feeling that the world and people are not real; individual feels distant

APPENDIX B

■ BIOPSYCHOSOCIAL ASSESSMENT

- Integrates patient's biological, psychological, and social aspects of his or her condition
- Biological factors are important in etiology and treatment of certain psychiatric disorders (e.g., schizophrenia)
- Social relationships and a history of developmental problems may leave certain individuals vulnerable to certain types of psychiatric illnesses
- Stressors may also precipitate individuals evolving certain psychiatric illnesses or having relapses of preexisting conditions
- Example of biopsychosocial history:
  - Childhood
    - Biological: development and health
    - Psychological: personality, temperament
    - Social: relationships within the family, school, and friends; any abuse or trauma
  - Adolescence
    - Biological: development and health
    - Psychological: personality, temperament
    - Social: relationships within the family, school, and friends; abuse or trauma; legal problems
  - Adult
    - Biological: development and health
    - Psychological: personality, temperament, religious affiliations, mood or behavioral problems
    - Social: relationships within any marriage, family, work, friends; legal problems; trauma or abuse; life stressors

Appendices

APPENDIX C

■ ERIKSON'S LIFE CYCLE STAGES

- **Trust vs. Mistrust**
  - Birth to 18 months
  - Infants are dependent and develop trust if they are appropriately cared after. Mistrust develops if their needs are not met.
- **Autonomy vs. Shame**
  - 18 months to 3 years
  - Children learn to communicate and make their own choices. If children do not learn to direct themselves, then they may become doubtful and resist attempting to do things by themselves.
- **Initiative vs. Guilt**
  - 3 to 6 years
  - Children learn to initiate actions and explore their environment; however, they may feel guilty for their attempts.
- **Industry vs. Inferiority**
  - 6 to 13 years
  - Children become industrious and enthusiastic to learn. If they feel inferior, then they lose interest in learning and creating.
- **Identity vs. Role Confusion**
  - 13 to 21 years
  - Adolescents develop a sense of unique identity; however, acceptance among others is also important. If they do not develop their own identity, then they may become confused about their direction in life.
- **Intimacy vs. Isolation**
  - 21 to 40 years
  - Adults must learn to balance the openness from intimacy with the loneliness created by isolation.
- **Generativity vs. Stagnation**
  - 40 to 60 years
  - Development of a positive outlook on one's role in life and society is important. If this fails, then one may go through life without concern for others.
- **Ego Integrity vs. Despair**
  - 60 years and older
  - Acceptance of life choices is necessary. If one does not accept his or her decisions, then regret may lead to despair.

■ FREUD'S PSYCHOSEXUAL DEVELOPMENT STAGES

- **Oral Stage**
  - Birth to 2 years
  - Infants gain satisfaction by oral stimulation through sucking and chewing.
- **Anal Stage**
  - 2 to 3 years
  - Children gain satisfaction through defecation or stool retention.
- **Phallic Stage**
  - 3 to 6 years
  - Children become curious about sex.
- **Latency Stage**
  - 6 to 12 years
  - Sexual desires are repressed.
- **Genital Stage**
  - Adolescents
  - Satisfaction of sexual urges is sought after.

■ PIAGET'S STAGES OF DEVELOPMENT

- **Sensorimotor**
  - Birth to 2 years
  - Infants begin learning through motor and sensory integration.
- **Preoperational**
  - 2 to 6 years
  - Children use language and imitation; they are not able to create continuous logical thought.
- **Concrete Operations**
  - 6 to 12 years
  - Children become able to produce logical thought through classification and relationships.
- **Formal Operations**
  - 12 years to adult
  - This stage involves logical reasoning, self-reflection, and the ability to process abstract ideas without dependence on concrete variables.

Appendix D

MEDICAL ETHICS AND COMMUNICATION

- **Beneficence:** Ethical responsibility of physician to act in the patient's best interest; however, a competent patient always has the ultimate decision.
- **Nonmaleficence:** First and foremost, "Do No Harm"; however, a competent patient always has the ultimate decision of whether to proceed with a treatment or not (e.g., patient may choose chemotherapy even though it may ultimately make the patient sick).
- **Confidentiality:** All communication between the physician and patient is private; however, the patient may waive the right to confidentiality to allow physician to discuss condition with family members or others; the physician may breach confidentiality when it is known to him or her that a third party may be subject to potential harm (e.g., homicidal plans), or if an adolescent has a serious condition that may be life-threatening or -altering, the physician may include the parents.
- **Competency and Decision-making Capacity:** Patient autonomy (an individual's right to make his or her own healthcare decisions) must be respected as long as the patient is competent or capable of making his or her own decisions; competency is assessed by a mental status exam (decisions not a result of delusion or hallucinations), and the patient is capable (e.g., not in an altered state of mind such as coma) of understanding the circumstances and of giving informed consent.
- **Full Disclosure:** Physician is responsible to fully disclose to the patient information regarding his or her condition; however, it is at the physician's discretion in what manner to disseminate the information so that the patient best understands it; if the family wishes to withhold information about a diagnosis, this does not outweigh the patient's right to know.
- **Informed Consent:** Decision-making process is a joint process between the physician and the patient; the patient is told the relevant information regarding the condition, interventions, risks, benefits, alternative treatments, and prognosis without treatment; all of the patient's questions are answered; the patient makes a final decision regarding intervention and to what degree; there is no third-party coercion.
- **Implied Consent:** In an emergency, the physician is allowed to intervene to care for a patient.
- **Oral Advance Directive:** Previous oral statements made by a now-incapacitated patient are used as a guide to direct treatment.
- **Written Advance Directive:** Consist of living wills (patient directs physician to withdraw or withhold life-sustaining treatment in terminal illness) and durable power of attorney (patient has assigned a surrogate to make decisions if patient is ever incapacitated).
- **Do-Not-Resuscitate Orders (DNRs):** Orders that are written at the patient's request that state cardiopulmonary resuscitation (CPR) should be withheld in the event of cardiac arrest; the patient's proxy may also make this request if the patient is incapacitated.

Appendices

APPENDIX E

EPIDEMIOLOGY AND BIOSTATISTICS

- **Sensitivity:** how accurate a test is at detecting patients who truly have a disease; high sensitivity correlates with a low false-negative; good for screening test because high accuracy in ruling OUT disease
- **Specificity:** how accurate a test is at detecting those without a disease; high specificity correlates with a low false-positive (does not falsely give positive result in patients without disease); remember negative in health or specific to health; good test for confirmation of diagnosis
- **Positive predictive value:** probability of truly having a disease given a positive test result; increases with prevalence
- **Negative predictive value:** probability of NOT having a disease given a negative test result

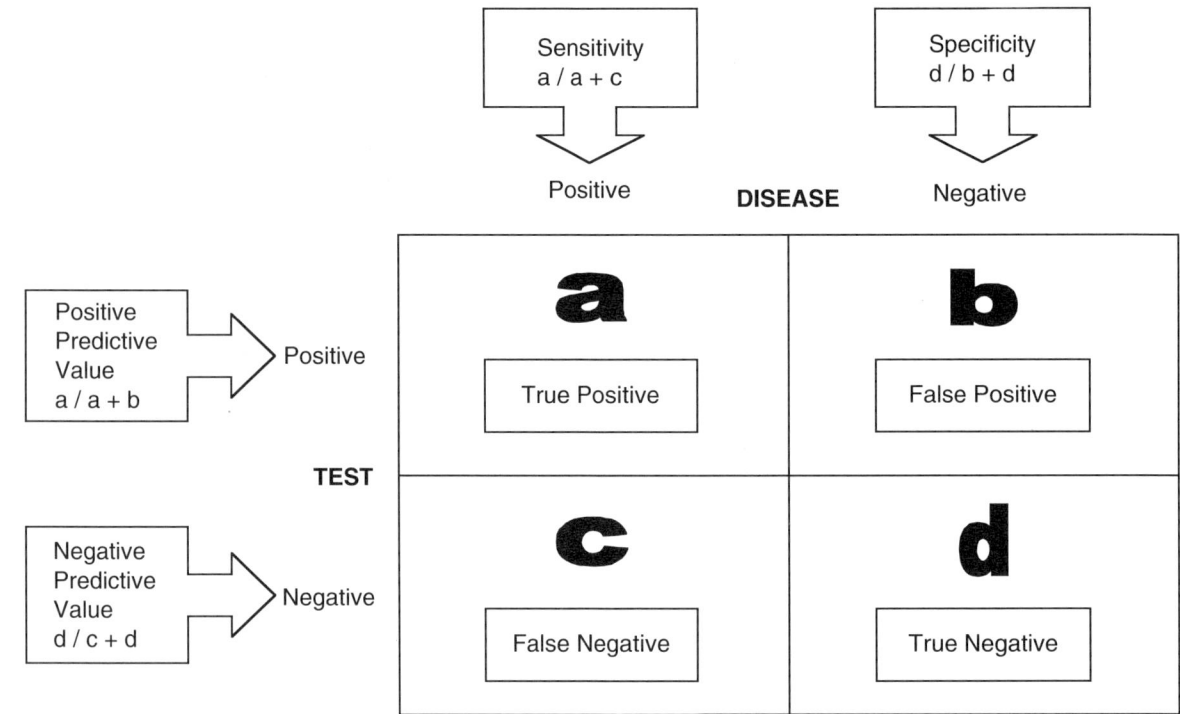

*Note that either a or d is in the numerator position.

- **Prevalence:** in a given unit of time, it is the number of individuals in a population with a particular condition
- **Incidence:** in a given unit of time, it is the number of new cases in a population
- **Precision:** reproducibility of a test
- **Accuracy:** correctness of a test's results/measurements

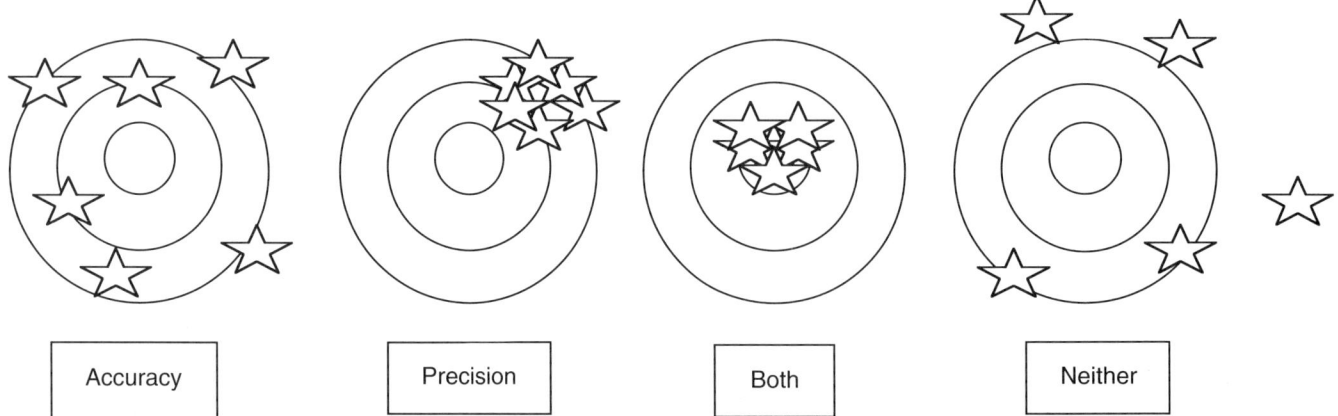

Appendices

- **Standard deviation:** (σ) measures variability of individuals within a population
- **Standard error of the mean:** (σ) / (square root of n the sample size); standard deviation of means in a sampling distribution; variability among means in future samples; standard error of the mean decreases as sample size increases
- **Bias:** error that leads to false conclusion in a study; secondary to method of patient selection, data collection and analysis, or method that conclusions are drawn
- **Meta-analysis:** combines results of several independent studies on one specific topic
- **Clinical trial:** experimental study that draws conclusions regarding treatments or procedures
- **Case-control study:** begins with absence (controls) or presence (cases) of a particular outcome, then study is conducted to determine risk factors (present in cases' histories but not present in controls' histories) for the outcome
- **Cohort study:** prospective study in which subjects are selected based on the characteristic that is suspected of being a risk factor for a particular disease or condition
- **H_1:** alternative hypothesis states that an association exists between the risk factor and disease
- **H_0:** null hypothesis states that no association exists between the risk factor and the disease

	Truth	
	H_1	H_0
Study Results H_1	**Power** $(1-\beta)$ Rejecting H_0 when you should as H_0 is false	α Type I error States there is effect when there is not (mistakenly accepted H_1 and rejected H_0)
H_1	β Type II error States there is not an effect when there is (mistakenly accepted H_0 and rejected H_1)	

INDEX

A
Abdominal pain, 44–45
Acetylcholinesterase inhibitors, 4
Acquired immunodeficiency disease. *See* HIV disease
Acting out, 114–115
ADD (attention deficit disorder), 86–88
Adolescent disorders, 86–99
Advance directives, 121
Affect, 6, 118
Agnosia, 4–5
Agoraphobia, 32–33, 82–83
AIDS. *See* HIV disease
Alcohol
    abuse of, 48–49, 70–71
    dependence on, 48–49
    intoxication from, 50–51
    withdrawal from, 2, 50
Alogia, 6
Altruism, 112–113
Alzheimer's disease, 4–5
Amenorrhea, 64–65
Amnesia
    dissociative, 68–69
    identity, 70–71
Amphetamines, 52–53
Anorexia nervosa, 64–65
Antisocial personality disorder, 22–23, 98
Anxiety disorders, 26–33
    generalized, 26–27
    OCD and, 28–29, 88
    panic disorder and, 32–33, 82–83
    PTSD and, 30–31, 68
Anxiolytics, 62–63. *See also* Benzodiazepines
Aphasia, 4–5
Apnea, sleep, 108–109
Apraxia, 4–5
Asperger's disorder, 92–93
Attention deficit disorder (ADD), 86–88
Autistic disorder, 90–91
Avoidant personality disorder, 24–25
Avolition, 6

B
Barbiturates
    intoxication from, 62
    withdrawal from, 2
Behavioral therapy, 102–105
Beneficence, 121
Benzodiazepines
    for alcohol withdrawal, 50
    for anxiety, 26
    dementia and, 4
    intoxication from, 62–63
    for OCD, 28
    for sleep disorders, 108
    withdrawal from, 2

Beta-blockers, 26, 28
Bias, 123
Binge eating, 64–67
Biopsychosocial assessment, 119
Biostatistics, 122–123
Bipolar disorders, 8–9, 16–17. *See also* Depression
Blocking thoughts, 6, 118
Body dysmorphic disorder, 40–41
Borderline personality disorder, 22–23
Bradyphrenia, 4
Brain tumor, 4
Broadcasting thoughts, 118
Bulimia nervosa, 66–67
Buspirone, 26, 28

C
Cannabis, 54–55
Carbon monoxide poisoning, 2
Case studies, 123
Cataplexy, 108–109
Catatonic behavior, 6–7
Child abuse, 72–73
Childhood disorders, 86–99
Circadian rhythms, 108–109
Clonidine, 60
Cocaine, 56–57
Cognitive impairment, 2–5
Cognitive therapy, 104–105
Cohort studies, 123
Collagen vascular disease, 4
Competency, 121
Compulsions, 28–29
Conditioning, 102–105
Conduct disorder, 98–99
Confidentiality, 121
Congestive heart failure (CHF), 4
Consent, 121
Conversion disorder, 36–37
Creutzfeldt-Jakob disease, 4
Cyclothymic disorder, 18–19

D
Decision-making capacity, 121
Delirium, 2–3
Delta sleep, 106–107, 110–111
Delusions
    definition of,
    paranoid, 6
    schizoaffective disorder and, 8–9
    schizophrenia and, 6–7
Delusional disorder, 10–11
Dementia, 4–5
    alcohol and, 50
    amnesia and, 68
Denial, 114–115
Depakote, 16
Dependence, 48–49. *See also* Substance abuse

Dependent personality disorder, 24–25, 114
Depersonalization, 58, 74–75
Depression. *See also* Bipolar disorders
    anorexia nervosa with, 64–65
    cyclothymic disorder and, 18–19
    dementia and, 4
    diagnosis of, 12–13
    dysthymic disorder and, 14–15
    major, 12–13, 64
    schizoaffective disorder and, 8–9
Derealization, 118
Desensitization, 104–105
Developmental stages, 120
Disclosure, 121
Disorganized behavior, 6–7
Displacement, 116–117
Dissociation, 116–117
Dissociative amnesia, 68–69
Dissociative disorders, 68–75
Dissociative identity disorder, 72–73
Disulfiram, 50
Donepezil, 4
Do-not-resuscitate (DNR) orders, 121
Dopamine, 6
Dream interpretation, 100–101
Dyspareunia, 78–79
Dysthymic disorders, 14–15

E
Eating disorders, 64–67
Echolalia, 6
Ecstasy, 58
Ego defenses, 112–116
Ejaculation, premature, 78–79
Encephalopathy, 4
Endocarditis, 4
Epidemiology, 122–123
Erectile disorder, 78–79
Erikson's life cycle, 120
Erotomania, 10–11
Ethics, 121
Exhibitionism, 80–81

F
Factitious disorder, 44–45
False beliefs, 6
Fetal alcohol syndrome, 50
Fetishism, 80–81
Flooding therapy, 26, 104–105
Flumazenil, 62
Fluoxetine. *See* Selective serotonin reuptake inhibitors
Folate deficiency, 4
Free association, 100–101
Freud, Sigmund, 100–101, 120
Frotteurism, 80
Fugue, dissociative, 70–71

G
Generalized anxiety disorder, 26–27. *See also* Anxiety disorders
Grandiose delusions, 10–11

H
Hallucinations
    defined, 118
    delirium and, 2–3
    delusional disorder and, 10–11
    dementia and, 4
    hypnagogic, 108–109
    LSD and, 58
    schizoaffective disorder and, 8–9
    schizophrenia and, 6–7
Hallucinogens, 58–59
Haloperidol, 2–3, 6
Head trauma
    amnesia and, 68
    delirium after, 2
    dementia after, 4
Hearing loss, 36
Histrionic personality disorder, 22–23
HIV disease
    anorexia nervosa and, 64
    dementia with, 4–5
    somatization disorder and, 34
Humor, 112–113
Huntington's disease, 4–5
Hydrocephalus, 4
Hyperactivity, 86–88
Hypercalcemia, 2
Hypercapnia, 2
Hyperparathyroidism, 4
Hypersomnia, 108–109
Hypnotics, 62–63. *See also* Barbiturates
Hypoactive sexual desire disorder, 78–79
Hypochondriasis, 38–39
Hypoglycemia, 2
Hypomania, 16, 18–19. *See also* Mania
Hyponatremia, 2

I
Ideas
    flight of, 118
    of reference, 20, 118
Identification, 116–117
Identity amnesia, 70–71
Identity disorder, 72–73
Illusion, 118
Implosion, 104–105
Impotence, 78–79
Impulsivity, 86–87
Informed consent, 121
Insight, 118
Insomnia, 108–109. *See also* Sleep disorders
Intellectualization, 116–117
Intoxication
    alcohol, 50–51
    amphetamine, 52–53
    anxiolytic, 62–63
    cannabis, 54–55
    cocaine, 56–57
    hallucinogen, 58–59
    opioid, 60–61
    sedative, 62–63
Ipecac, 66

J
Jealousy
    delusional disorder and, 10–11
    personality disorders and, 20
    projection and, 116–117
Jet lag, 109–110
Judgment, 118

K
K complexes, 106–107

L
Laxative abuse, 66–67
Learning disorders, 50
Life cycle stages, 120
Lithium, 16
Lorazepam, 2
LSD, 58–59
Lupus erythematosus, 34
Lysergic acid diethylamide (LSD), 58–59

M
Major depressive disorder, 12–13, 64. *See also* Depression
Maleficence, 121
Malingering, 46–47
Mania
    bipolar disorders and, 16–17
    cyclothymic disorder and, 18–19
    hypo, 16, 18–19
    schizoaffective disorder and, 8–9
Marijuana, 54–55
Masochism, 80
MECP2 gene, 94
Medical ethics, 121
Memory impairment
    alcohol and, 50
    delirium and, 2–3
    dementia and, 4–5
    sedatives and, 62–63
Meningitis, 4
Mescaline, 58
Meta-analysis, 123
Methadone, 60
Methaqualone, 62
Methylenedioxyamphetamine (MDMA), 58
Methylphenidate, 108–109
Modanfinil, 108
Modeling, 102–103
Mood, 118
Mood disorders, 12–19. *See also specific types, e.g.,* Depression
Multiple personality disorder, 72–73
Multiple sclerosis, 4, 34
Munchausen's syndrome, 44–45

N
Naloxone, 60
Narcissistic personality disorder, 22–23
Narcolepsy, 108–109
Negative symptoms, 6
Neologisms, 118
Neurosyphilis, 4
Nightmares, 110–111
Nonmaleficence, 121
Non-REM sleep, 106–107
Null hypothesis, 123
Numbness, 36–37
Nystagmus
    alcohol and, 50
    sedatives and, 62–63

O
Obsessive-compulsive disorder (OCD), 28–29, 88
Obsessive-compulsive personality disorder, 24–25
Opioids, 60–61
Oppositional defiant disorder, 96–97
Orgasmic disorder, 78–79

P
Pain disorder, 42–43
Pain syndromes
    factitious, 44–45
    somatization disorder and, 34–35
Panic disorder, 32–33, 82–83
Paralysis, 36–37
Paranoia
    amphetamines and, 52
    delusions and, 10–11
    hallucinogens and, 58
    schizophrenia with, 6–7
Paranoid personality disorder, 20–21
Paraphilias, 80–81
Parasomnias, 110–111
Parkinson's disease, 4–5
Pedophilia, 80
Personality disorder(s), 20–25
    antisocial, 22–23, 98
    avoidant, 24–25
    borderline, 22–23
    cluster A, 20–21
    cluster B, 22–23
    cluster C, 24–25
    dependent, 24–25, 114
    histrionic, 22–23
    narcissistic, 22–23
    obsessive-compulsive, 24–25
    paranoid, 20–21
    schizoid, 20–21
    schizotypal, 20–21
Phobia, 32–33, 64, 82–85
Piaget's developmental stages, 120
Pick's disease, 4–5
Pill-rolling tremor, 4
Polysomnography, 106–107
Positive symptoms, 6–7

Post-traumatic stress disorder (PTSD), 30–31, 68
Predictive value, 122
Premature ejaculation, 78–79
Projection, 116–117
Pseudodementia, 4
Pseudoneurologic symptoms, 34–35
Psychoanalysis, 100–101
Psychosexual disorders, 76–79
Psychotherapies, 100–105
Psychotic disorders, 6–11
PTSD. *See* Post-traumatic stress disorder
Purging, 64–67

R
Rationalization, 114–115
Reaction formation, 114–115
Reference, ideas of, 20, 118
Regression, 114–115
REM sleep, 106–107, 110–111
Repression, 112–113
Rett's disorder, 94–95

S
Sadism, 80
Schizoaffective disorder, 8–9
Schizoid personality disorder, 20–21
Schizophrenia, 6–7
Schizophreniform disorder, 6–7
Schizotypal personality disorder, 20–21
Sedatives, 62–63. *See also* Barbiturates
Seizures
　alcohol withdrawal and, 50
　amphetamines and, 52–53
　conversion disorder and, 36
　factitious, 44–45
　sedatives and, 62
Selective serotonin reuptake inhibitors (SSRIs)
　for anorexia nervosa, 64–65
　for anxiety, 26
　for bulimia nervosa, 66–67
　for depersonalization disorder, 74–75
　for depression, 12
　for OCD, 28
　for pain disorder, 42–43
Sensitivity, 122
Sexual aversion disorder, 78–79
Sexual dysfunction, 34–35, 78–79

Sexual response, 76–77
Sleep disorders, 106–111
　alcohol and, 50
　dementia and, 4
　depression and, 12–13
　dyssomnias and, 108–109
　parasomnias and, 110–111
Sleep stages, 106–107
Sleep terrors, 110–111
Sleepwalking, 110–111
Social phobia, 64, 84–85
Somatic delusions, 10–11
Somatization disorder, 34–35
Somatoform disorders, 34–43
Specificity, 122
Speech impairments
　autism with, 90–91
　dementia with, 4–5
　schizophrenia with, 6–7
Splitting, 114–115
Spongiform encephalopathy, 4
SSRIs. *See* Selective serotonin reuptake inhibitors
Standard deviation, 123
Starvation, 66
Statistics, 122–123
Stress
　conversion disorder and, 36–37
　depersonalization disorder and, 74–75
　dissociative fugue and, 70–71
Sublimation, 112–113
Substance abuse, 48–63
　alcohol, 48–51
　amphetamine, 52–53
　anxiolytic, 62–63
　cannabis and, 54–55
　cocaine, 56–57
　defined, 48
　delirium from, 2
　dependence and, 48–49
　dissociative fugue and, 70–71
　hallucinogens and, 58–59
　opioid, 60–61
　pain disorder and, 42–43
　sedative, 62–63
Sundowning
　delirium and, 2–3
　dementia and, 4–5
Suppression, 112–113

Syphilis, 4
Systemic lupus erythematosus, 34

T
Tacrine, 4
Tegretol, 16
Thiamine deficiency
　alcohol abuse and, 50
　delirium from, 2
　dementia from, 4
Thyroid disorders
　delirium from, 2
　dementia from, 4
Tics, 88–89
Token therapy, 104–105
Tourette's disorder, 88–89
Transference, 100–101
Tranvestism, 80–81
Trazodone, 108
Tremor, pill-rolling, 4

U
Undoing, 116–117
Urinary tract infections, 2

V
Vaginismus, 78–79
Vascular dementia, 4–5
Vision loss, 36–37
Vitamin B12 deficiency, 4
Voyeurism, 80

W
Wernicke-Korsakoff syndrome, 50
Wilson's disease, 4
Withdrawal syndromes
　alcohol, 2, 50
　amphetamine, 52
　anxiolytic, 62
　barbiturate, 2
　benzodiazepine, 2
　cocaine, 56
　opioid, 60
　sedative, 62

Z
Zaleplon, 108
Zolpidem, 108–109